Begad M. Samy
Fatma Kamel
Hala Abdulhady

Effect Of Training On Diastolic Function In Male Volleyball Players

D1796836

Begad M. Samy
Fatma Kamel
Hala Abdulhady

Effect Of Training On Diastolic Function In Male Volleyball Players

Athlete' Heart Vs Hypertrophic Cardiomyopathy

LAP LAMBERT Academic Publishing

Impressum/Imprint (nur für Deutschland/only for Germany)
Bibliografische Information der Deutschen Nationalbibliothek: Die Deutsche Nationalbibliothek verzeichnet diese Publikation in der Deutschen Nationalbibliografie; detaillierte bibliografische Daten sind im Internet über http://dnb.d-nb.de abrufbar.
Alle in diesem Buch genannten Marken und Produktnamen unterliegen warenzeichen-, marken- oder patentrechtlichem Schutz bzw. sind Warenzeichen oder eingetragene Warenzeichen der jeweiligen Inhaber. Die Wiedergabe von Marken, Produktnamen, Gebrauchsnamen, Handelsnamen, Warenbezeichnungen u.s.w. in diesem Werk berechtigt auch ohne besondere Kennzeichnung nicht zu der Annahme, dass solche Namen im Sinne der Warenzeichen- und Markenschutzgesetzgebung als frei zu betrachten wären und daher von jedermann benutzt werden dürften.

Coverbild: www.ingimage.com

Verlag: LAP LAMBERT Academic Publishing GmbH & Co. KG
Heinrich-Böcking-Str. 6-8, 66121 Saarbrücken, Deutschland
Telefon +49 681 3720-310, Telefax +49 681 3720-3109
Email: info@lap-publishing.com

Approved by: Egypt, Ain Shams University, Diss., 2012

Herstellung in Deutschland (siehe letzte Seite)
ISBN: 978-3-8454-2449-1

Imprint (only for USA, GB)
Bibliographic information published by the Deutsche Nationalbibliothek: The Deutsche Nationalbibliothek lists this publication in the Deutsche Nationalbibliografie; detailed bibliographic data are available in the Internet at http://dnb.d-nb.de.
Any brand names and product names mentioned in this book are subject to trademark, brand or patent protection and are trademarks or registered trademarks of their respective holders. The use of brand names, product names, common names, trade names, product descriptions etc. even without a particular marking in this works is in no way to be construed to mean that such names may be regarded as unrestricted in respect of trademark and brand protection legislation and could thus be used by anyone.

Cover image: www.ingimage.com

Publisher: LAP LAMBERT Academic Publishing GmbH & Co. KG
Heinrich-Böcking-Str. 6-8, 66121 Saarbrücken, Germany
Phone +49 681 3720-310, Fax +49 681 3720-3109
Email: info@lap-publishing.com

Printed in the U.S.A.
Printed in the U.K. by (see last page)
ISBN: 978-3-8454-2449-1

Contents

INTRODUCTION...1

AIM OF THE WORK...7

REVIEW OF LITERATURE........................…......9

CHAPTER 1: CARDIORESPIRATORY PHYSIOLOGY..9

CHAPTER 2: BASIC PRINCIPLES OF EXERCISE
TRAINING AND CONDITIONING..........................18

CHAPTER 3: ATHLETE'S HEART.........................26

CHAPTER 4: EXERCISE PRESCRIPTION AND
PROGRAM...................................…...........59

SUBJECTS AND METHODS...............................75

RESULTS ....…......107

DISCUSSION.................................…......135

SUMMARY AND CONCLUSION.........................159

RECOMMENDATIONS......................................163

REFRENCES...165

List of figures

No	Title	Page
1	Classification of sports.	30
2	Schematic of Doppler diastolic transmitralflow velocity.	35
3	Pulsed Doppler recordings of transmitral filling (panelA) and color M-mode Doppler echocardiography (panel B).	36
4	Clinical criteria used to distinguish non obstructive HCM from athlete's heart.	43
5	Echocardiography of an international cyclist and a patient with morphologically mild hypertrophic cardiomyopathy.	45
6	Causes of sudden death in young competitive athlete.	55
7	Echocardiographic test in left lateral position.	78
8	Echocardiography in supine position in our study.	78
9	Echocardiography showing Cardiac chambers diameters and systolic function from our study.	80
10	Echocardiography showing diastolic function from our study.	82
11	Color M-mode Doppler showing diastolic function.	83

12	Zan 600 ergospirometer from the apparatus manual.	**85**
13	Zan 600 control unit with connected mask, ergo flow sensor and power supply.	**86**
14	Applying ECG leads and the respiratory mask in our study	**88**
15	A player performing the test in our study	**88**
16	A player performing the test in our study	**89**
17	Vo2 max report taken from one of our subjects	**90**
18	A player performing static stretching to right quadriceps Muscle	**94**
19	A player performing static stretching to leftt hamstring and calf muscles	**95**
20	A player performing static stretching to left adductor group muscles taken from our study	**95**
21	Strengthening exercise program for shoulder abductors muscle taken from our study	**101**
22	Strengthening exercise program for shoulder flexors muscle taken from our study	**102**
23	Strengthening exercise program for the biceps brachii muscle taken from our study	**102**
24	Strengthening exercise program for the triceps muscle taken from our study	**103**
25	Strengthening exercise program for wrist extensors taken from our study	**103**
26	Strengthening exercise program for the quadriceps muscle taken from our study	**104**
27	Strengthening exercise program for the adductors and abductors of the hip taken from our study	**104**
28	Highly significant difference in (IVST), (PWT). And significant difference in (LVEDD). And no significant difference in (LVMI) and (LVESD).	**119**

29	Highly significant difference in (SV), and significant difference in (FS) and (EF) before and after training	**120**
30	Highly significant difference in (Vp), and no significant differences in E/A ratio and (DT) before and after trainin	**122**
31	No significant difference Between Serum cardiac Troponin T before and after training	**123**
32	Highly significant difference in Vo2 max before and after training	**124**
33	Correlation between age and (Vp) **before training**	**125**
34	Correlation between BMI (DT) before training	**126**
35	Correlation between BMI and Vo2 max before training	**127**
36	Correlation between Vo2 max and Vp before training	**128**
37	Correlation betweenVo2max and E/A ratio after training	**129**
38	Correlation between Vo2 max and Vp after training	**130**
39	Correlation between CTnT and DT after training	**131**
40	Correlation between change in VO2 max and change in Vp	**132**
41	Correlations between change in VO2 max and changes in E/A ratio	**133**
42	Correlations between change in VO2 max and change in DT	**134**

List of tables

No	Title	Page
1	Differential diagnosis between athlete's heart and HCM	41
2	Normal Vo2 max values in ml/kg/min in non athletes.	86
3	Vo2 max in ml/kg/min in some athletes.	87
4	demographic data	107
5	Vital data	108
6	Description of echocardiographic cardiac structure.	110
7	Echocardiographic Systolic function	111
8	Echocardiographic cardiac Diastolic function.	112
9	Serum cardiac troponin T	112
10	Maximal O2 consumption of the muscles (Vo2 max)	113
11	Description of echocardiographic cardiac structure after training	114
12	Description of cchocardiographic cardiac Systolic function after training	115
13	Description of Echocardiographic cardiac Diastolic function after training.	116

14	Serum cardiac troponin T after training.	116
15	Maximal O2 consumption of the muscles (Vo2 max) after training.	117
16	Comparison between echocardiographic cardiac structure before and after training	118
17	Comparison between echocardiographic cardiac systolic function before and after training.	120
18	Comparison between echocardiographic cardiac Diastolic function before and after training.	121
19	Comparison between serum troponin level before and after training.	123
20	Comparison between Maximal O2 consumption of the muscles (Vo2 max) before and after training.	124

Introduction

Long-term athletic training is associated with cardiac changes including increased left ventricular (LV) cavity dimension, wall thickness, and calculated mass that have been extensively studied and are commonly described as "athlete's heart" (**Spirito et al., 1994).**

In general, studies have proven that athletes participating in purely endurance sports such as long distance running and tennis are subject to chronic increases in cardiac preload which causes increase in stroke volume through increasing end diastolic volume, while those participating in purely resistance sports such as weightlifting and body-building tend to develop a large increase in LV wall thickness which increase stroke volume through decreasing end systolic volume **(Fagard 2003).**

Volleyball has been recently classified as a moderate static and high dynamic sport, therefore involving a combination of resistance and endurance training **(Dzudie et al., 2007).**

Differentiating physiologic from pathologic LV hypertrophy is an important challenge, as highly trained

1

competitive athletes without apparent heart disease can develop markedly thickened ventricular walls that may resemble hypertrophic cardiomyopathy **(Chee et al., 2005).**

Among the criteria used to differentiate between the pathological LV hypertrophy and the adaptive hypertrophy of athletes, is diastolic filling. Several authors **(Kingue et al., 2001)** have reported a normal diastolic filling in physiological hypertrophic states, whereas pathologic LV hypertrophy such hypertrophic cardiomyopathy or aortic stenosis affects diastolic filling and associated with diastolic dysfunction, characterized by impaired ventricular relaxation and filling which manifest on echocardiographic assessment as Doppler velocity abnormalities **(Ommen and nishimura, 2003).** In contrast with the situation in patients with cardiovascular diseases, left ventricular hypertrophy associated with athletic training is likely to be a benign or beneficial adaptation which does not impact on ventricular relaxation in the same manner as pathological hypertrophy **(louise et al., 2005).**

Endurance performance depends mainly on the oxidative energy-yielding capacity of the body. Good aerobic performance needs good respiratory function, good circulatory transport, and a high level of oxidative enzyme capacity in the skeletal muscles. A crucial part of this system is the athlete's heart. Otherwise, any higher level of endurance performance is almost impossible without well-adapted cardiac function **(Claessens et al., 2004).**

A commonly used method to investigate endurance capacity is the measurement of the maximal oxygen uptake by spiroergometry. It can therefore be assumed that spiroergometrically measured maximal oxygen consumption will correlate with various attributes of the athlete's heart as an important determinant of aerobic performance **(Kneffel et al., 2007).**

VO2 max has been defined as: "the highest rate of oxygen consumption attainable during maximal or exhaustive exercise" As exercise intensity increases, so does oxygen consumption. However, a point is reached where exercise intensity can continue to increase without the associated rise in oxygen consumption (**Wilmore and Costill 2005).**

3

The troponin complex is located on the thin filament of striated muscle which include skeletal and cardiac muscle. It consists of the proteins troponin T, troponin I and troponin C, and plays a central role in the regulation of muscle contraction. The amino acid sequences of cardiac troponin T (cTnT) and troponin I (cTnI) are sufficiently dissimilar and therefore detectable by monoclonal antibody– based assays (Braunwald et al., 2002). Troponin C is not used clinically because both cardiac and smooth muscle share troponin C isoforms. Therefore cardiac troponin T isoform (cTnT) and the cardiac troponin I isoform (cTnI) measured in serum or plasma are highly sensitive and specific markers of acute myocardial injury, and are recommended for the diagnosis of acute myocardial infarction **(Lowbeer et al., 2007).**

However, several diseases other than acute myocardial injury can be associated with serum cardiac troponin T (cTnT) elevations. **(Jeremias et al., 2005).** These elevations may arise from various causes which are not fully understood. Other causes include sepsis, hypotension, supraventricular tachycardia, cardiac contusion, cardiac transplantation and ingestion of sympathomimetic drugs or chemotherapy. In dialysis patients

4

and in heart failure (HF) patients, cTnT correlates positively with increased left ventricular mass, suggesting an association between pathological left ventricular hypertrophy (LVH) and elevated serum cTnT concentrations **(Duman et al., 2005).**

Recently, Baseline serum cTnT concentrations were not elevated in healthy professional football players with physiological eccentric LVH. These findings suggest that cTnT leakage from hearts with an enlarged left ventricle associated with systematic training is very unlikely in healthy athletes practicing intermittent high intensity team sports. Therefore the association between cTnT and left ventricular hypertrophy as shown previously in patients with heart failure **(Lowbeer et al., 2004)** is not explained by LVH per se, but more likely by a combination of LVH and the disease state where a variety of pathophysiologic mechanisms such as capillary-cardiomyocyte mismatch, myocardial fibrosis and changes in myocardial metabolism may predispose patients to myocardial damage **(Lowbeer et al., 2007).**

Aim of the work

The aim of this work is :-

To study the ability of diastolic function measured by echocardiography to reflect changes in endurance as assessed by Vo2 max in response to combined strengthening and endurance training in male volleyball players.

To detect any subclinical cardiac changes by mean of serum cardiac troponin T in male volleyball players.

Cardiorespiratory Physiology

The cardiorespiratory system consists of the heart, lungs, and blood vessels. The purpose of this system is for the delivery of oxygen and nutrients to the cells as well as the removal of metabolic waste products in order to maintain the internal equilibrium **(Holly and Shaffrath, 2001).**

I-Cardiac Function

a) Heart Rate

Normal resting heart rate (HRrest) is approximately 60–80 beats/min. With the onset of dynamic exercise, HR increases in proportion to the relative workload. The maximal HR (HRmax) decreases with age, and can be estimated in healthy men and women subtracting age from 220. There is considerable variability in this estimation for any fixed age with a standard deviation of 10 beats/min **(Rupp, 2001; Holly and Shaffrath, 2001).**

b) Stroke Volume

Stroke volume (SV) is the amount of blood ejected from the left ventricle in a single beat. SV is equal to the difference between end diastolic volume (EDV) and end systolic volume

9

(ESV). Greater diastolic filling (preload) will increase SV. Factors that resist ventricular outflow (afterload) will result in a reduced SV.

During endurance exercise, SV increases curvilinearly with the work rate until it reaches near maximum at a level equivalent to approximately 50% of aerobic capacity. Thereafter, SV starts to plateau and further increases in workload do not result in increased SV primarily owing to reduced filling time during diastole. **(Darren et al., 2008).**

SV is also affected by body position, with SV being greater in the supine or prone position and lower in the upright position. Static exercise (weight training) may also cause a slight decrease in SV owing to increased intrathoracic pressure **(Goodman et al., 2005).**

c) Cardiac Output

Cardiac output (Q) is the amount of blood pumped by the heart each minute. Resting cardiac output in both trained and sedentary individuals is approximately 4–5 L/min; however, during endurance exercise maximal cardiac output can reach 20 L/min. During dynamic exercise, cardiac output increases with increasing exercise intensity by increases in SV and HR; however, increases in cardiac output beyond 40–50% of VO2max are accounted for only by increases in HR **(Darren et al., 2008).**

d) Blood Flow

At rest, 15–20% of the cardiac output is distributed to the skeletal muscles with the remainder going to visceral organs, the brain and the heart; however, during any type of exercise, 85–90% of the cardiac output is selectively delivered to working muscles. Myocardial blood flow may increase four to five times with exercise, whereas blood supply to the brain is maintained at resting levels. The difference between the oxygen content of arterial blood and the oxygen content of venous blood is termed the arteriovenous oxygen difference (a-vO2 Diff.). It reflects the oxygen extracted from arterial blood by the tissues. At rest the oxygen extraction is approximately 25%, but at maximal exercise the oxygen extraction can reach 75% **(Darren et al., 2008).**

11

e) Venous return

Venous return is maintained and/or increased during dynamic exercise by contracting skeletal muscles which act as a pump. And by contraction of smooth muscle around the venules, increasing the pressure on the venous side. Also diaphragmatic contraction during exercise creates lowered intrathoracic pressure, facilitating blood flow **(Rupp, 2001; Holly and Shaffrath, 2001).**

f) Blood Pressure

Blood pressure (BP) is the driving force behind blood flow. Systolic blood pressure (SBP): SBP increases linearly with increasing work intensity, by 8–12 mm-Hg per metabolic equivalent (MET), where 1 MET = 3.5 mLO-2/kg/min. Maximal values typically reach 190 to 220 mm-Hg. Maximal SBP should not be greater than 260 mm-Hg. Diastolic blood pressure (DBP) either remains unchanged or only slightly increases with exercise **(Rupp, 2001).**

Failure of SBP to rise or decreased SBP with increasing work rates or a significant increase in DBP is an abnormal response to exercise and indicates either severe exercise

12

intolerance or underlying cardiovascular disease. At similar oxygen consumptions, HR, SBP, and DBP are higher during arm work than during leg work **(Darren et al., 2008).**

II- Pulmonary Ventilation

Pulmonary ventilation (Ve) is the volume of air exchanged per minute, and generally is approximately 6 L/min at rest in an average sedentary adult male; however, at maximal exercise, Ve increases 15-to 25-fold over resting values. During mild to moderate dynamic exercise Ve increases primarily by increasing tidal volume, but during vigorous activity increases in the respiratory rate are the primary way Ve increases **(Franklin, 2001).**

Generally, increases in Ve are directly proportional to an increase in oxygen consumption (VO2) and carbon dioxide produced (VCO2); however, at a critical exercise intensity (usually 47–64% of the VO2max in healthy untrained individuals and 70–90% VO2max in highly trained individuals predominantly dynamic sports), Ve increases disproportionately relative to the VO2, paralleling an abrupt increase in serum lactate and VCO2. This is called the anaerobic (ventilatory) threshold (AT) **(Franklin, 2001).**

AT signifies the onset of metabolic acidosis during aerobic exercise, and traditionally has been determined by serial measurements of blood lactate. It can be noninvasively determined by assessment of expired gases during exercise testing, specifically Ve and VCO2. AT signifies the peak work rate or oxygen consumption at which the energy demands exceed circulatory ability to sustain aerobic metabolism **(Franklin, 2001).**

III-Maximal Oxygen Consumption

The most widely recognized measure of cardiopulmonary fitness is the aerobic capacity, or VO2max. This variable is defined physiologically as the highest rate of oxygen transport and use that can be achieved at maximal physical exertion **(Franklin, 2001).**

Effects Of Exercise On Cardiovascular System

The effects of regular exercise on the cardiovascular system can be grouped into changes that occur at rest, during submaximal exercise and during maximal work **(Rupp, 2001).**

1) Changes at Rest

- Heart rate (HR) decreases likely secondary to decreased sympathetic tone, increased parasympathetic tone, and a decreased intrinsic firing rate of the SA node.

- SV increases secondary to increased myocardial contractility.

- Cardiac output is unchanged at rest.

- Oxygen consumption does not change at rest .

2) Changes at Submaximal Work

Submaximal work is defined as a workload during which a steady state is achieved.

- HR decreases at any given workload owing to the increased SV and decreased sympathetic drive.

- SV increases owing to increased myocardial contractility.

- Cardiac output does not change significantly for a fixed workload; however, the same cardiac output is generated with a lower HR and higher SV.

- Oxygen consumption does not change significantly since oxygen requirement is the similar for a fixed workload.

- Lactate levels are decreased owing to metabolic efficiency and increased lactate clearance rates **(Rupp, 2001)**.

3) Changes at Maximal Work

- Maximal heart rate (HRmax) does not change with exercise training.

- SV increases owing to increased contractility and/or increased heart size.

- Maximal cardiac output increases owing to increased SV.

- Maximal oxygen consumption (VO2max) increases owing to increased SV and A-vO2 difference owing to improved ability of the mitochondria to use oxygen **(Rupp, 2001)**.

Effect of Detraining on cardiovascular system

The changes induced by regular exercise training generally are lost after 4–8 weeks of detraining. If training is reestablished, the rate at which the training effects occur do not appear to be faster **(Rupp, 2001)**.

Effect of Overtraining on cardiovascular system

Overtraining refers to a condition usually induced after prolonged heavy exercise over an extended period of time. Symptoms of overtraining may include sudden decline in quality of work or exercise performance, extreme fatigue, elevated HR at rest, early onset of blood lactate accumulation, altered mood states, unexplained weight loss, Insomnia and injuries related to overuse. Overtraining may require weeks to months of complete rest in order to recover **(Rupp, 2001).**

Basic principles of exercise training and conditioning

Introduction

Regular physical activity is an important component of a healthy lifestyle. Increases in physical activity and cardio respiratory fitness have been shown to reduce the risk of death from coronary heart disease as well as from all causes. There is increasing evidence showing that regular participation in moderate-intensity physical activity is associated with health benefits, even when aerobic fitness remains unchanged. To reflect this evidence, the Centers for Disease Control and Prevention (CDC) and the American College of Sports Medicine (ACSM) are now recommending that every adult accumulate 30 min or more of moderate intensity physical activity on most—and preferably all—days of the week. Those who follow these recommendations will experience many of the health-related benefits of physical activity, and if they are interested in achieving higher levels of fitness, will be ready to do so **(Whaley and Kaminsky, 2001)**

18

Metabolic Energy Systems

At rest, a 70-kg human has an energy expenditure of about 1.2 kcal/min with less than 20% of resting energy expenditure attributed to skeletal muscle; however, during intense exercise, total energy expenditure may increase 15–25 times above resting values, resulting in a caloric expenditure between 18 and 30 kcal/min. Most of this increase is used to provide energy to the exercising muscles, which may increase energy requirements by a factor of 200 **(Demaree et al, 2001).**

Role Of Adenosine Triphosphate

The energy used to fuel biological processes comes from the breakdown of adenosine triphosphate (ATP), specifically from the chemical energy stored in the bonds of the last two phosphates of the ATP molecules. When work is performed, the bond between the last two phosphates is broken, producing energy and heat.

The limited stores of ATP in skeletal muscles can fuel approximately 5–10 s of high-intensity work. Therefore, ATP must be continuously resynthesized from adenosine diphosphate (ADP) to allow exercise to continue. Muscle fibers contain three metabolic pathways for producing ATP which are creatine phosphate, rapid glycolysis, and aerobic oxidation **(Rupp, 2001).**

Creatine Phosphate System

When limited stores of ATP are nearly depleted during high-intensity exercise (5–10 s), the creatine phosphate (CP) system transfers a high-energy phosphate from CP to rephosphorylate ATP from ADP. Since it involves a single reaction, this system can provide ATP at a very rapid rate; however, as there is a limited supply of CP in the muscle the amount of ATP that can be produced is also limited.

There is enough CP stored in skeletal muscle for approximately 25 s of high-intensity work. Therefore, the ATPCP system will last for about 30 s (5 s for the stored ATP,and 25 s for CP). This will provide energy for activities such as sprinting and weight lifting. The CP system is considered an anaerobic system since oxygen is not required **(Knuttgen ,2003).**

Rapid Glycolysis (Lactic Acid System)

Glycolysis uses carbohydrate, primarily muscle glycogen as a fuel source. When glycolysis is rapid, it is capable of producing only a few ATP without involvement of oxygen. Lactic acid is also produced as a product of this reaction. The accumulation of excessive amounts of lactic acid in muscle tissue is associated with fatigue. The lactic acid system produces enough energy to last approximately 1–2 min before the accumulation of excessive lactic acid would produce fatigue. It would fuel activities such as middle distance sprints (400, 600 and 800 m runs). Although glycolysis is considered an anaerobic pathway, it can readily participate in aerobic metabolism when oxygen is available, and it is considered the first step in the aerobic metabolism of carbohydrate **(Kraemer, 2003).**

Aerobic Oxidation System

The final metabolic pathway for ATP production combines two complex metabolic processes, the Krebs cycle and the electron transport chain. This system resides in the mitochondria. It is capable of using carbohydrates,fat, and small amounts of protein to produce energy (ATP) during exercise through a process called oxidative phosphorylation. During exercise this pathway uses oxygen to completely metabolize the carbohydrates to produce energy (ATP) leaving only carbon dioxide and water as by-products. The aerobic oxidation system is complex, and thus requires 2–3 min to adjust to a change in exercise intensity; however, it has an almost unlimited ability to regenerate ATP, limited only by the amount of fuel and oxygen that is available to the cell.

Maximal oxygen consumption, also known as VO2 max, is a measure of the power of the aerobic energy system and is generally regarded as the best indicator of aerobic fitness **(Wilmore, 2003).**

Fuel Usage During Exercise

All the energy-producing pathways are active during most exercise; however, different types of exercise place greater demands on different pathways. The contribution of the anaerobic pathways (CP system and glycolysis) to exercise energy metabolism is inversely related to the duration and

22

intensity of the activity. The shorter and more intense the activity, the greater the contribution of anaerobic energy production; whereas the longer the activity and the lower the intensity, the greater the contribution of aerobic energy production. In general, carbohydrates are used as the primary fuel at the onset of exercise and during high-intensity work; however, during prolonged exercise of low to moderate intensity (longer than 30 min), a gradual shift from carbohydrate toward an increasing reliance on fat as a substrate occurs. The greatest amount of fat use occurs at about 60% of maximal aerobic capacity (VO2max) (**Demaree et al, 2001; Rupp, 2001**).

Muscle Physiology

Classification Of Muscle Fibers

Skeletal muscle cells are organized into motor units, and each unit is controlled by a single motor (efferent) neuron with its cell body located in the gray matter of the spinal cord. Each motor neuron's single axon emerges as a part of a motor nerve trunk and continues all the way to the particular skeletal muscle fibers it innervates (**Knuttgen , 2007**).

23

The muscle fibers of a single motor unit are homogeneous and are classified broadly as Type I (slow-twitch) or Type II (fast-twitch) with differing functional and metabolic characteristics. The type of muscle fiber recruited to perform a specific activity depends on intensity and duration of exercise.

Most muscles contain both fast-twitch and slow-twitch muscle fibers; however, the ratio of fast-twitch to slow twitch muscle fibers varies in an individual. The ratio also differs within the same muscle from one individual to another **(Humphrey, 2001).**

Type I (Slow-Twitch) Muscle Fibers

Type I fibers are those that resist fatigue and thus are recruited for lower intensity, longer duration activities. Sedentary persons have approximately 50% Type I, and this distribution is generally equal throughout the major muscle groups of the body. Endurance athletes have a greater percentage of Type I fibers thought to be the result of genetic predisposition **(Humphrey, 2001).**

Type II (Fast-Twitch) Muscle Fibers

Type II fibers are muscle fibers that can generally generate a great deal of force very rapidly. These fibers are

24

recruited when a person is performing high-intensity activities. These fibers can produce large amounts of tension in a very short time period, but the accumulation of lactic acid from anaerobic glycolysis causes them to fatigue quickly. Type II fibers are subdivided into Type IIa and IIb fibers. Type IIa fibers: Type IIa fibers represent a transition type of fiber. While these fibers are capable of generating a moderately large amount of force, they also have some aerobic capacity, although not as much as the Type I fibers. These fibers represent a logical and necessary bridge between the two types of muscle fibers allowing one to meet the energy demands for a variety of physical tasks. Type IIb fibers: Type IIb fibers are the classic fast twitch fibers that are predominately anaerobic since they rely on energy sources intrinsic to the muscle. **(Humphrey, 2001).**

Resistance training stimulates synthesis of muscle proteins and can lead to hypertrophy, whereas endurance training causes a partial phenotype transformation from fast to slow fibre type **(Wackerhage et al., 2005).**

Athlete's Heart

In contemporary sports medicine, the term 'athlete's heart' is used to describe the characteristic enlargement (hypertrophy) of the myocardium in response to repeated exercise stimuli **(Maron, 1996).**

The principle features of 'athlete's heart' include cardiac enlargement to allow for increased maximal stroke volume (SV) and cardiac output, adaptations that drive the increase in oxygen delivery in the trained state since no training effect is evident in maximal heart rate (HRmax) **(Whyte et al., 2007).**

The phenomenon of athlete's heart is now so widely accepted that it is often used as a benchmark for characterizing elite-level athletes. Associated with this is the widely held concept that different exercise training modalities produce divergent patterns of cardiac hypertrophy in athletes. This sports-specific hypothesis was first presented by Joel Morganroth and colleagues in the 1970s who hypothesized that the cardiac morphological adaptation observed in athletes corresponded with the nature of the hemodynamic stimulus imposed on the ventricles during repeated exercise bouts.

26

Endurance training purportedly leads to an eccentric form of cardiac hypertrophy, principally characterized by increased left ventricular (LV) cavity dimension, and thus LV mass (LVM), as a consequence of prolonged repetitive volume overload. In contrast, strength training is supposedly associated with a concentric form of hypertrophy where increased ventricular wall thickness, with no change in cavity size. This has been commonly referred to as the "Morganroth hypothesis" **(Naylor et al., 2008).**

Classification of Sports from the cardiovascular point of view

Sports are classified according to their type, dynamic (isotonic) or static (isometric), and to their intensity, low, moderate or high. Briefly, dynamic exercise involves changes in muscle length and joint movement with rhythmic contractions that develop a relatively small intramuscular force, and static exercise induces development of a large intramuscular force with little or no change in muscle length or joint movement **(Mitchell et al., 2005)**.

27

These two types of exercises should be thought of as the two opposite poles of a continuum, with most physical activities involving both static and dynamic components. For example, distance running has low static and high dynamic demands; body building has principally high static and low dynamic demands, and rowing or canoeing have both high static and dynamic demands **(Barbier et al., 2006)**.

Other sports classifications mainly proposed by sports medicine physicians are based upon the energetic, i.e., aerobic and anaerobic, demand of the sport concerned. The terms dynamic and static exercise characterize physical activity on the basis of the mechanical action of skeletal muscles involved and differ from the terms aerobic and anaerobic exercise. For example, high-intensity static exercise is performed with anaerobic metabolism, whereas high-intensity dynamic exercise lasting for more than several minutes is performed mainly with aerobic metabolism. However, some dynamic exercises, such as sprinting or jumping, are performed primarily with anaerobic metabolism **(Barbier et al., 2006)**.

28

The classification of sport is based on peak static and dynamic components achieved during competition. It should be noted, however, that higher values may be reached during training. The increasing dynamic component is defined in terms of the estimated percent of maximal oxygen uptake (MaxO2) achieved and results in an increasing cardiac output. The increasing static component is related to the estimated percent of maximal voluntary contraction (MVC) reached and results in an increasing blood pressure load. The lowest total cardiovascular demands (cardiac output and blood pressure) are shown in green and the highest in red this is shown in figure 1.

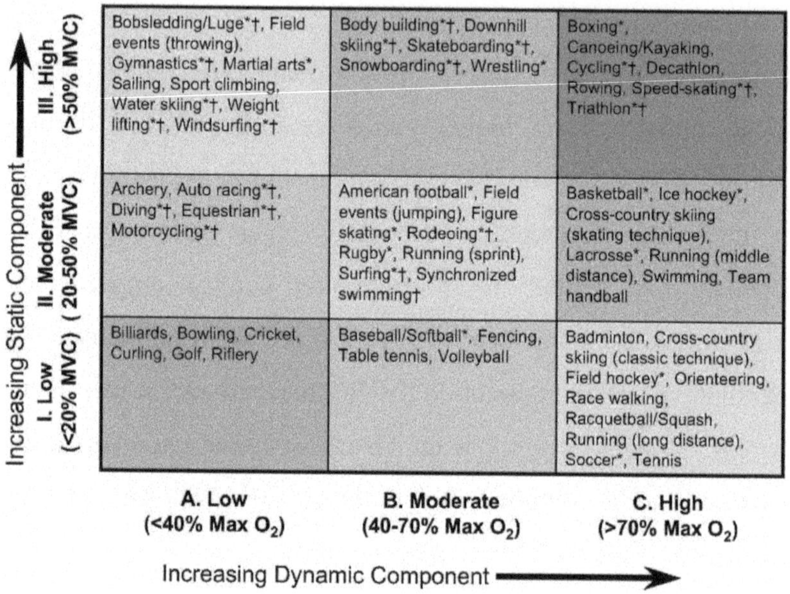

		A. Low (<40% Max O_2)	B. Moderate (40-70% Max O_2)	C. High (>70% Max O_2)
III. High (>50% MVC)		Bobsledding/Luge*†, Field events (throwing), Gymnastics*†, Martial arts*, Sailing, Sport climbing, Water skiing*†, Weight lifting*†, Windsurfing*†	Body building*†, Downhill skiing*†, Skateboarding*†, Snowboarding*†, Wrestling*	Boxing*, Canoeing/Kayaking, Cycling*†, Decathlon, Rowing, Speed-skating*†, Triathlon*†
II. Moderate (20-50% MVC)		Archery, Auto racing*†, Diving*†, Equestrian*†, Motorcycling*†	American football*, Field events (jumping), Figure skating*, Rodeoing*†, Rugby*, Running (sprint), Surfing*†, Synchronized swimming†	Basketball*, Ice hockey*, Cross-country skiing (skating technique), Lacrosse*, Running (middle distance), Swimming, Team handball
I. Low (<20% MVC)		Billiards, Bowling, Cricket, Curling, Golf, Riflery	Baseball/Softball*, Fencing, Table tennis, Volleyball	Badminton, Cross-country skiing (classic technique), Field hockey*, Orienteering, Race walking, Racquetball/Squash, Running (long distance), Soccer*, Tennis

Increasing Static Component →

Increasing Dynamic Component ⟶

Figure 1: Classification of sports. This classification based on peak static and dynamic components achieved during competition. MVC: maximal voluntary contraction. Adopted from Mitchell et al., 2005.

Echocardiographic adaptations in athlete's heart

In case of physiological cardiac hypertrophy, according to Laplace's law and in order to reduce the increased wall tension induced by LV dilatation, LV wall thickness must increase. Thus, in accordance with this theory, the greatest increase in LV wall thickness must occur in the largest dilated LV. However , most endurance sports are associated with a large LV diastolic diameter, they are not always associated with the same increase in wall thickness **(Spirito et al., 1994).**

Thus, other factors and mainly training specificity may also be involved in these adaptations. Sports-specific adaptive cardiac structural changes are somewhat controversial. The two different classic morphological forms of athlete's heart, strength trained and endurance-trained, previously proposed by Morganroth hypothesis are not really confirmed **(Pluim et al., 2000).**

Briefly, and according to the theory by Morganroth athletes involved in sports with a high dynamic component are presumed to demonstrate eccentric LV hypertrophy, with a great LVEED and a proportional increase in wall thickness, in response to volume overload, whereas strength-trained athletes are presumed to develop concentric LV hypertrophy, with unchanged LVEED and increased wall thickness, in response to pressure overload **(Barbier et al., 2006).**

31

In accordance with data by **(Pluim et al., 2000).** It actually appears that most of highly trained athletes develop an LV fair combination of cavity dilatation and increased wall thickness. However, ventricular dilatation slightly predominates in endurance athletes, whereas the increased wall thickness slightly predominates in static ones **(Thomas and Douglas, 2001).** The association of dynamic and static training sessions, whatever the sport practiced, may partly explain these results. **(Barbier et al., 2006).**

Myocardial Functions

Functional adaptations, which seem to precede structural myocardial adaptations, have been described in trained subjects, however, the question of whether athlete's cardiac hypertrophy is a purely physiological phenomenon or should be considered a risk factor like cardiac hypertrophy induced by pathologic, causes as hypertrophic cardiomyopathy, hypertension or aortic stenosis, is still under debate **(Pluim et al., 1999).**

Systolic LV function most often expressed as the fractional shortening (FS), is usually normal in athlete's heart whatever the sports practiced **(Vinereanu et al., 2001).**

32

Myocardial tissue Doppler assessment of systolic function has recently confirmed these results **(Erol et al., 2002).** In professional cyclists, however, a decreased resting systolic function has been noted **(Abergel et al., 2004).**

Some studies have also shown that right cardiac function is normal in athlete's heart **(Erol et al., 2002).** In trained subjects, despite the increased LV mass and whatever the sports practiced, cardiac diastolic function is normal **(Saito et al., 2004)** or increased in comparison with untrained subjects **(Barbier et al., 2006).**

Diastolic function

Diastole is the summation of processes by which the heart loses its ability to generate force and shorten and returns to its precontractile state. The two principal processes responsible are relaxation and passive pressure–volume properties of the ventricle. However, the diastolic properties of the ventricle are complex and multifactorially determined and are related to the speed and synchrony of myocardial relaxation and inactivation, loading conditions, viscoelasticity, heart rate, atrial function, and ventricular interaction **(Hoit, 2007).**

Echocardiographic Assessment Of Diastolic Function

During diastole, there is an initial phase of rapid transmitral flow as the mitral valve opens and the left ventricle relaxes; this early filling phase results in a peak in the transmitral flow profile referred to as the E wave. The early filling phase is followed by a period of slow filling called diastasis, during which the slowing of left ventricular relaxation and the rise in left ventricular diastolic pressure result in a decrease in transmitral flow velocity. A late phase of rapid filling occurs with atrial contraction, resulting in a second peak in the transmitral flow profile referred to as the A wave **(Moller et al., 2000).**

The isovolumic relaxation time (IVRT) is the interval between the closing of the aortic valve and the opening of the mitral valve, when left ventricular relaxation begins but before left ventricular volume begins to increase. The diastolic deceleration time (DDT) is the interval between the peak early diastolic filling velocity (the peak of the E wave) and the end of the E wave, when diastasis begins. The IVRT and DDT are prolonged in patients with impaired left ventricular relaxation and shortened in patients with restrictive physiology as shown in figure 2 **(Hoit, 2007).**

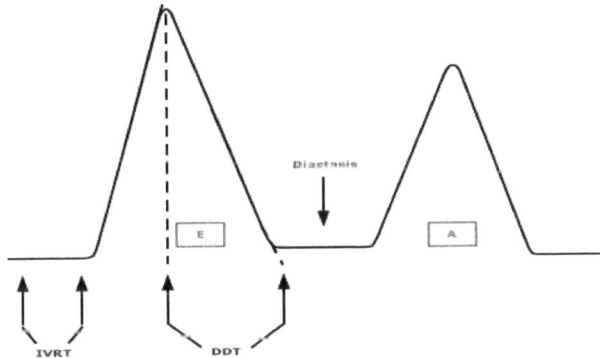

Figure 2: Schematic of Doppler diastolic transmitral flow velocity.(IVRT) isovolumic relaxation time, (DDT) diastolic deceleration time, (E) peak E and (A) peak A.

Echocardiographic M-mode color Doppler flow propagation velocity (Vp) measures spatial and temporal propagation of early diastolic flow, and its velocity in the LV cavity. Vp is an index of ventricular relaxation that does not pseudonormalize and has been shown to be independent constant of isovolumic relaxation this is shown in figure 3 (**Tumuklu et al., 2007**).

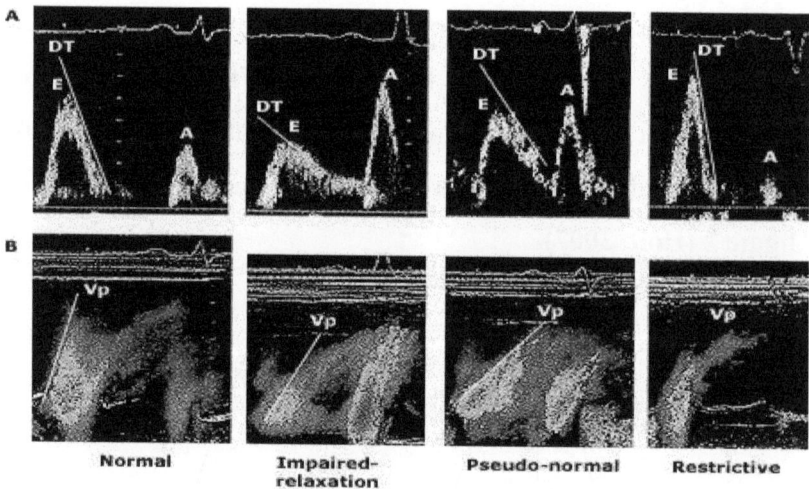

Normal   **Impaired-relaxation**   **Pseudo-normal**   **Restrictive**

Figure 3: Pulsed Doppler recordings of transmitral filling (panel A) and color M-mode Doppler echocardiography (panel B).

Doppler echocardiography (panel B) are methods for evaluating left ventricular (LV) diastolic function. In a normal filling pattern, the mitral E-wave deceleration time (DT) is 140 to 240 ms and the M-mode flow propagation velocity (Vp) is $\geq$ 45 cm/s). In diastolic dysfunction with impaired relaxation the DT is prolonged $\geq$240 ms and Vp is normal or reduced (<45 cm/s). In a pseudonormal filling pattern the DT may be normal or prolonged, but the Vp is <45 cm/s. In diastolic dysfunction with a restrictive filling, the DT is <140 ms and the Vp is normal or <45 cm/s. Patients with a myocardial infarction who have a restrictive or pseudonormal pattern have an increased incidence of left ventricular dilation and cardiac death (**Moller et al., 2000**).

Effects of exercise training on cardiac (diastolic) Function

As pointed out by Libonati in 1999 , the ability of cardiac function to meet the excess demands for increased cardiac output during exercise is largely dependent upon the ability to increase LV filling. It follows, given the progressive decline in filling time with exercise, that transmitral diastolic pressure gradients must increase during results from enhanced diastolic suction. If acute bouts of exercise are associated with enhanced diastolic filling, one may assume that repetitive bouts cause physiological adaptation which favours enhanced indices of diastolic function. Balanced against this is the possibility that training-induced ventricular hypertrophy, albeit physiological in nature and extent, may be associated with ventricular stiffening which compromises diastolic function, as seen in the clinical arena **(Green et al., 2006).**

Cross-sectional studies and meta-analyses suggest that the resting E/A ratio is unchanged, or significantly (although modestly) increased in athletes compared with controls, with all values being within the normal range. These data, although consistent, should not be over interpreted; early filling velocity (E) is usually not different between athletes and controls, indicating that decreased atrial filling velocity (A) is responsible for the presence of enhanced E/A in athletes. This, in turn, is likely a reflection of the reduction in resting heart rate and consequently prolonged atrial filling period in trained individuals **(Green et al., 2006).**

Color M-mode flow propagation velocity (Vp), a spatiotemporal index of LV relaxation and relatively insensitive to alterations in left atrial pressure and heart rate, was impaired after a period of detraining in athletes, who nonetheless exhibited residual LV hypertrophy relative to matched controls.

38

Resumption of training in the athletes further increased LV mass, but was associated with improved propagation velocity, a finding unlikely to be related to changes in heart rate **(Hoit, 2007).**

This raises the hypothesis that diastolic function may be normal in the athletes who exhibit ventricular hypertrophy so long as the training stimulus is extant; resolution of exercise-induced ventricular remodeling following cessation of training in elite endurance athletes may lag, with possible consequences for diastolic function **(Hoit, 2007).**

Thus, in comparison with pathologic cardiac hypertrophy , the physiological cardiac hypertrophy of athlete's heart is not accompanied by disturbances of resting diastolic parameters **(Pluim et al., 2000).**

Hypertrophic cardiomyopathy Vs athlete's heart

Hypertrophic cardiomyopathy (HCM) is the commonest cause of sudden cardiac death in the young, especially the young athletes **(Maron, 2005)**. The fact that young athletes, especially elite athletes, often have enlarged hearts has been known before HCM was described, Tung in China noticed in 1930 a markedly enlarged heart in an otherwise healthy athlete, employed in one of the departments of his hospital, during a routine physical examination. This finding led to the study of 46 healthy athletes nearly half of whom showed definite cardiac enlargement, which he reported in 1934 **(Tung, 1934) (Cheng, 2007)**.

When HCM becomes one of the commonest causes of sudden cardiac death in the young athletes, it becomes imperative to distinguish it from athlete's heart. Athlete's heart is a physiological and benign adaptation to training, whereas HCM is a pathological and potentially malignant process with risk for sudden cardiac death. Fortunately, such a differentiation is possible nowadays **(Cheng, 2009)**

Differentiation between HCM and athlete's heart

The following table shows the difference between athletes heart and HCM in different points as quoted from **Cheng, 2009.**

Table 1: Differential diagnosis between athlete's heart and HCM

	Athlete's heart	HCM
Family history	-	+
LV hypertrophy	Symmetrical	Asymmetrical
LV thickness	< 13 mm	>15 mm
LV cavity	>55 mm	< 45 mm
LA enlargement	Mild	Moderate
Mitral E/A ratio	>1	< 1
Tissue Doppler	High velocity	Low velocity
Tissue strain rate	Normal	Reduced
PeakO2 consumption	>50 mi/min/kg	< 45 ml/min/kg
N-terminal pro-BNP	Normal	Elevated
Stopping training	Regression	No regression
Genetic testing	Negative	Positive

HCM: hypertrophic cardiomyopathy, LV: left ventricular, LA: left atrial, LVOT: left ventricular outflow tract, O2: oxygen and N-Terminal pro-BNP: amino terminal pro-brain natriuretic peptide.

1. Family history

HCM is a familial disease. In the fascinating historical article by **Watkins et al.** published in 1992, the authors reported the fate of different members of the original family reported in by **Teare in 1958**. Four of the six family members of the same generation had HCM and one died; four of the next generation had HCM from which one died and one was resuscitated from an out-of-the-hospital cardiac arrest. There is, of course, no such family history in the athletes with the athlete's heart **(Watkins et al., 1992).**

2. Left ventricular hypertrophy

In athlete's heart, left ventricular hypertrophy is symmetrical while in HCM, the hypertrophy of the left ventricle is asymmetrical **(Maron et al., 1981)**, with the anterior ventricular septum being the most thickened segment. Furthermore, contiguous left ventricular walls often show strikingly different thicknesses, often with abrupt transition between adjacent segments **(klues et al., 1995).**

3. Left ventricular wall thickness

On the basis of examination of 947 athletes, Spirito in 1994 found that left ventricular thickness of more than13 mm

42

extremely uncommon. In HCM, the left ventricular wall thickness is 15 mm. modest segmental wall thickening between 13 and 15 mm is a gray zone (figure 4), which raises the differential diagnosis between physiological left ventricular hypertrophy in athlete's heart and mild HCM. However, this can usually be resolved with other noninvasive testing **(Maron, 2002)**.

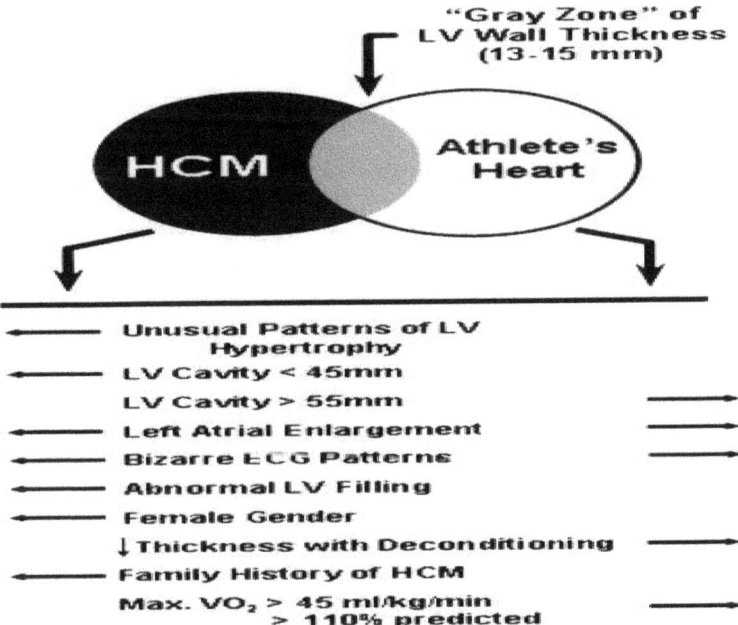

Figure 4:. Clinical criteria used to distinguish non obstructive HCM from athlete's heart when maximal LV wall thickness is within shaded gray area of overlap, consistent with both diagnoses. Adapted from Maron et al with permission of the American Heart Association. Copyright 1995.

4. Left ventricular cavity size

Athlete's heart has not only increased left ventricular wall thickness but also increased left ventricular end diastolic cavity size of about 55 mm , on the other hand, HCM is characterized by a small left ventricular cavity size of about 45 mm in end-diastole as shown in figure 5 **(Cheng, 1990)**. Moreover, the enlarged left ventricular cavity in athlete's heart maintains its normal elliptical shape with a normal position of the mitral valve without mitral regurgitation. On the other hand, the distribution of left ventricular hypertrophy in HCM is asymmetrical and heterogeneous, and the left ventricular geometry is usually distorted . Distortion of the mitral valve apparatus in HCM often results in mitral regurgitation with a resultant mitral regurgitant murmur. In athlete's heart there is usually no heart murmur; if a murmur is present, it is usually a systolic ejection murmur heard over the pulmonary area due to increased cardiac output **(Pelliccia et al., 2000).**

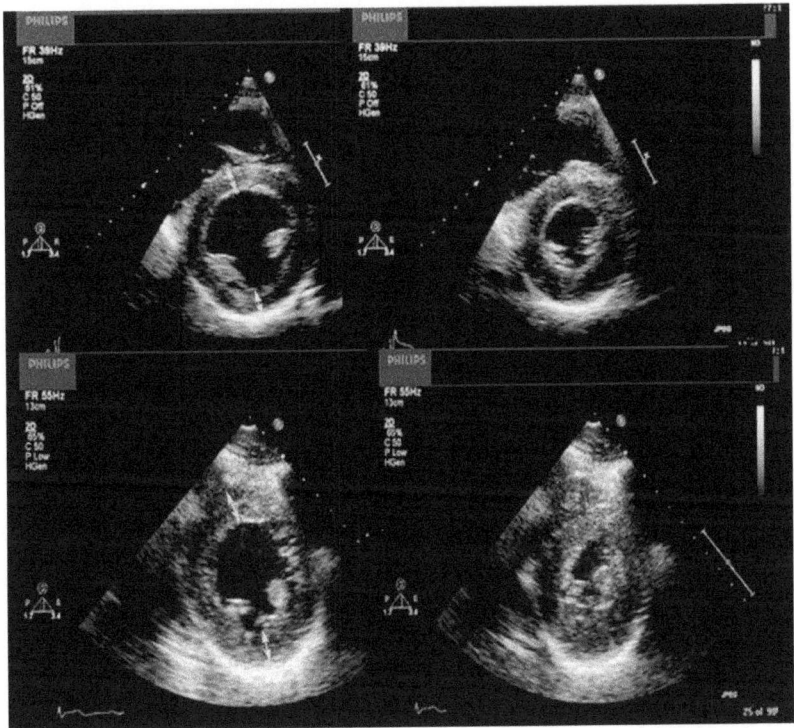

Figure 5: Echocardiography of an international cyclist (top) and a patient with morphologically mild hypertrophic cardiomyopathy (bottom). Showing a left ventricular wall thickness of 13 mm (arrows) in both individuals. However, note the athlete has an enlarged left ventricular cavity (60 mm) when compared with the patient with HCM (44 mm).

5. Left atrium

Atrial fibrillation is uncommon in athlete's heart, and similar in prevalence to the general population **(Maron, 2002)**. On the other hand, atrial fibrillation is the most common sustained arrhythmia in HCM and the result of left atrial enlargement **(pelliccia et al., 2005)**.

Mild left atrial enlargement is relatively common in competitive athletes and represents a physiological adaptation to exercise conditioning, largely without adverse clinical consequences **(pelliccia et al., 2005)**. Left atrial enlargement is moderate in HCM and represents the consequence of impaired left ventricular compliance and/or mitral regurgitation. It has a prognostic significance, particularly relevant to the identification of patients at risk for death related to congestive heart failure **(Nistri et al., 2006)**.

6. Left ventricular outflow tract obstruction

Left ventricular outflow tract obstruction is absent in athlete's heart but present in HCM. Although left ventricular outflow tract obstruction may not be apparent in every patient

46

with HCM at rest, it can usually be brought by exercise, various maneuvers or pharmacological agents **(Cheng, 2001).** Two thirds of patients with non obstructive HCM have latent left ventricular outflow tract obstruction **(Vagilo et al., 2008).**

7. Mitral E/A ratio

In athlete's heart the left ventricular diastolic function is well preserved, and thus provides an important point of distinction from HCM. Therefore, Doppler echocardiography shows a normal filling pattern with the early peak of transmitral flow velocity (E) increased and the late atrial (A) peak decreased, resulting in an E/A ratio greater than 1 (1.7 ± 0.4) **(Griffet et al., 2007).**

In contrast, patients with HCM, including those with mild left ventricular hypertrophy that could possibly be confused with athlete's heart, consistently show abnormal Doppler diastolic indexes of left ventricular filling. Typically the E/A ratio is inverted . However, a normal diastolic left ventricular filling pattern is not particularly helpful, because it is compatible with either athlete's heart or HCM **(pelliccia et al., 2004).**

47

8. Tissue Doppler

Tissue Doppler imaging is a relatively sensitive method for the assessment of cardiac function that provides direct, local measurements of myocardial velocities throughout the cardiac cycle **(Krieg et al., 2007).**

In athlete's heart, tissue Doppler imaging shows a high myocardial velocity in both systole and diastole, in contrast, low left ventricular systolic and diastolic velocities are found in HCM **(Rajiv et al., 2004).** Reduced myocardial velocities have even been observed in mutation carriers before the development of left ventricular hypertrophy in HCM **(D'Andrea et al., 2006)**

9. Tissue strain rate

Strain rate imaging derived from tissue Doppler imaging is a newly developed echocardiographic modality and an emerging technique to quantify regional myocardial function and assess both systolic and diastolic functions **(Richard et al., 2007).** The strain rate was significantly reduced in patients with HCM **(Cheng, 2008).**

10. Peak oxygen consumption

Peak oxygen consumption (VO2 max) values during exercise in elite athletes usually range between 55 and 70 ml/kg/min and exceed predicted maximum values by as much as 50% .In contrast, patients with HCM have impaired left ventricular filling during exercise, which prevents the augmentation of stroke volume required to achieve a high cardiac output on exercise. This test is particularly useful in individuals in the "gray zone" **(Sharma et al., 2000)**. However, (VO2 max) has certain limitations when assessing strength athletes, because the latter may have values that may overlap with patients with HCM **(Anastasakis et al., 2005)**.

11. N-Terminal pro-brain natriuretic peptide

Amino terminal pro-brain natriuretic peptide (NT-proBNP) is now routincly used to detect congestive heart failure. NTproBNP, which was previously reported to be usually normal in healthy athletes, was recently reported to be elevated in HCM, thus, in active athletes presenting with ambiguous left ventricular hypertrophy, abnormal NT-proBNP levels indicate HCM, whereas normal values are inclusive **(Godon et al., 2009)**

12. Stopping training

Because left ventricular hypertrophy is a physiological consequence of athletic training, it should regress after stopping of training. This was predicted in 1951 by White, who said "Cardiac enlargement, apparently largely dilatation, found in some athletes during their period of intensive sport, may subside when the athletic life is given up" **(White, 1951),** Even left ventricular hypertrophy in highly trained Olympic athletes may show a substantial reduction (by 2–5 mm) after a 3-month de-conditioning period **(Maron et al., 1993).**

A longitudinal study in 40 elite male athletes after a long-term de-conditioning period (1–13 years; mean, 5.6±3.8) showed significant reduction in cavity size and normalization of left ventricular wall thickness **(Pelliccia at al., 2002).** On the contrary, no such regression in left ventricular wall thickness would be expected to occur in patients with HCM following cessation of exercise training **(Pelliccia at al., 2005).**

13. Genetic testing

Mutation analysis for 8 commonest HCM causing genes is now commercially available. Unfortunately, due to the heterogeneity of HCM, a negative test does not exclude the possibility that an individual's HCM is due to a mutation in a gene that was not tested. Therefore, although a positive test result in an athlete can resolve the diagnostic ambiguity between athlete's heart and HCM, a negative test may be a false negative **(Maron et al., 2004).**

Prevalence of HCM in athletes

Although HCM is the commonest cause of sudden cardiac death in young athletes **(Maron, 2005),** the prevalence of HCM in elite athletes is extremely low in both the Western world **(Basavarajaiah et al., 2008)** and China **(Ma et al., 2007)**

Of the 3500 athletes studied by **Basavarajaiah et al., 2008**, only 3 (0.09%) athletes had left ventricular morphology that could have been regarded as being consistent with HCM. However, all had an E/A ratio greater than 1; E/A ratio in HCM is less than 1.

51

In China, 351 elite athletes were examined between June 2005 and July 2005 and none showed any evidence of HCM **(Ma et al., 2007).** A note of caution, however, is in order here. There is a racial difference in ECG and echocardiographic changes between white and black athletes, as was reported recently **(Magalski at al., 2008).**

Black athletes tend to show higher incidence of ECG abnormalities **(Magalski at al., 2008)** and greater magnitude of left ventricular hypertrophy **(Basavarajaiah et al., 2008)** than white athletes. Therefore, extrapolation of conclusions derived from white athletes may generate a false diagnosis of HCM in black athletes **(Basavarajaiah et al., 2008).**

It is vitally important to distinguish physiologic left ventricular hypertrophy in athletes (athlete's heart) from pathologic left ventricular hypertrophy in HCM. This is particularly pertinent nowadays in view of the tragic, unexpected and often highly publicized sudden cardiac death of top-level athletes reported by the news media **(Cheng, 2009).**

52

Whereas HCM is the commonest cause of sudden cardiac death in the young athletes, its occurrence in elite athletes is extremely rare. Although there are many similarities between athlete's heart and HCM, distinguishing the two is possible in the majority of cases. Genetic testing will play a major role in the future in the definitive resolution of this very important differential diagnosis **(Cheng, 2009).**

Cardiovascular risks of sports

Sudden Death in Athletes

Sudden death occurring in athletic individuals was once regarded as a mysterious and undefined syndrome; however, a voluminous body of literature defining the cardiovascular and other causes of these catastrophes has been assembled over the last several years **(Maron, 2003).** Nevertheless, the perception persists in the community that it is counterintuitive for young and highly trained high school, college, or professional athletes to unknowingly harbor potentially lethal cardiovascular disease susceptible to sudden and unexpected death **(Pelliccia et al., 2005).**

53

Mechanisms of sudden death

Sudden death in young athletes usually occurs on the athletic field and is related to physical activity, in the absence of prior symptoms **(Maron, 2003).** Indeed, the incremental risk for sudden death in adolescents and young adults is significantly higher (ie, 2.8-fold greater) when associated with vigorous physical exertion during competitive sports. Exercise acts as a trigger for lethal ventricular tachyarrhythmias, given the susceptibility imposed by underlying (and usually unsuspected) cardiac disease **(Corrado et al., 2003).**

Causes of sudden death

A number of largely congenital and often clinically silent cardiovascular diseases have been causally linked to sudden deaths in young trained athletes in autopsy surveys (Figures 6).

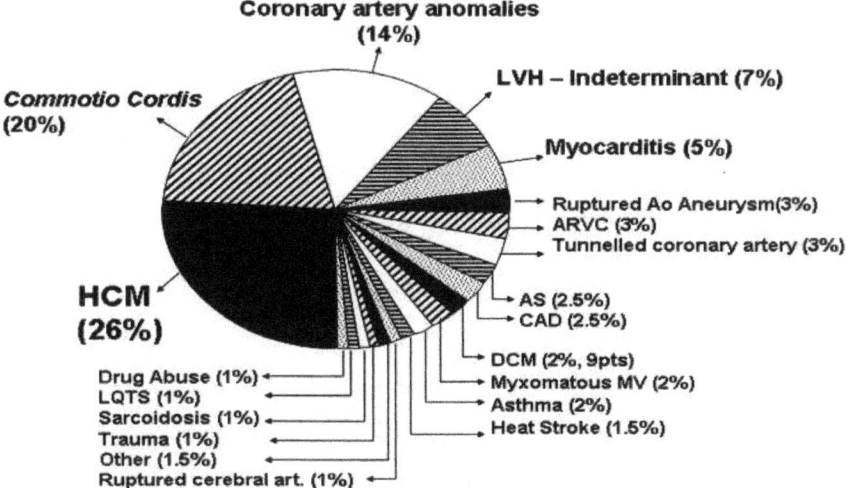

Figure 6: Causes of sudden death in young competitive athletes, as reported to the Minneapolis Heart Institute Foundation national registry. (AS) aortic stenosis, (CAD) coronary artery disease, (DCM) dilated cardiomyopathy, (LQTS) long-QT syndrome, (ARVC) arrhythmogenic right ventricular cardiomyopathy, (LVH) LV hypertrophy and (MV) mitral valve.

In the United States, hypertrophic cardiomyopathy (HCM) has been consistently reported to be the single most common cardiovascular cause, accounting for approximately one third of the deaths **(Burke et al., 1991).** Indeed, 3 recent and highly visible sudden deaths or cardiac arrests that occurred in US professional athletes were each caused by HCM, as well as a notable sudden death in a Cameroon soccer player which was diagnosed as HCM that occurred during a televised international match **(Maron, 2005).**

The second most frequent cause of these deaths in athletes is commotio cordis followed by congenital coronary artery anomaly of wrong sinus origin (most commonly, left main coronary artery origin from right sinus of Valsalva) **(Basso et al., 2000).** Diagnosis requires a high index of suspicion in young athletes presenting with exertional chest pain and/or syncope, because 12-lead or exercise ECG abnormalities suggestive of ischemia are usually absent **(Basso et al., 2000).**

A diverse array of other diseases each accounts for a much smaller proportion (5% to 8%) of the cardiovascular deaths in young athletes (Figure 4) These include myocarditis, valvular heart disease (aortic stenosis and myxomatous mitral valve disease), premature atherosclerotic coronary artery disease, dilated cardiomyopathy, arrhythmogenic right ventricular cardiomyopathy (ARVC), or aortic dissection and rupture (usually associated with Marfan syndrome) **(Youngblood, 2005).**

56

Sudden cardiovascular death may occur in a wide variety of more than 30 competitive athletic disciplines, most commonly basketball and American football in the United States and soccer in Europe, intense sports that also have high participation levels **(Van Camp et al., 1995).** These sudden death events also occur much more frequently in males (by 9:1); young women are probably less frequently affected because of their lower overall participation rates and absence from sports such as football, also blacks account for a disproportionate number of sports related sudden deaths owing to previously undiagnosed HCM **(Barry et al., 2006).**

Extreme LV remodeling evident in some highly trained athletes has intuitively raised a concern of whether such exercise-related morphological adaptations are always innocent. One longitudinal echocardiographic study reported incomplete reversal of extreme LV cavity dilatation with deconditioning; substantial chamber enlargement persisted in 20% of retired and deconditioned former elite athletes after 5 years **(Pelliccia et al., 2002).** There is no evidence at present showing that athlete's heart remodeling leads to long term disease progression, cardiovascular disability, or sudden cardiac death. The possibility that persistence of extreme remodeling after prolonged and intensive conditioning will ultimately convey deleterious cardiovascular consequences to some athletes is perhaps unlikely but at this time cannot be excluded with certainty **(Barry et al., 2006).**

Exercise Prescription And Program

The American College of Sports Medicine (ACSM) recommendations For cardiorespiratory Endurance Training Mode recommend that the best improvements in cardiorespiratory endurance occur when large muscle groups are engaged in rhythmic aerobic activity. And that various activities can be incorporated into an exercise program to increase enjoyment and improve compliance.

Endurance training improves oxygen transport and leads to a more efficient use of oxygen by way of an increased density of capillaries, myoglobin concentration, number and size of mitochondria, and greater activity of oxidative enzymes within the mitchondria **(Reilly, 2007)**.

Appropriate activities include—walking, jogging, cycling, rowing, stair climbing, aerobic dance (aerobics), water exercise, and cross-country skiing **(Franklin et al, 2000)**.

Intensity

The ACSM recommends that exercise intensity prescribed within a range of 70–85% of HRmax, 50–85% of VO2max, or 60–80% of max METs, or HR reserve (HRR).

1. Owing to the variability in estimating HRmax from age, whenever possible use an actual HRmax from a graded exercise test.

2. Lower intensities (40–50% of VO2max) elicit a favorable response in individual with very low fitness levels **(Franklin et al, 2000).**

Rating of perceived exertion (RPE) may be used with HR for regulating intensity.

1. ACSM recommends an intensity that will elicit an RPE within a range of 12–16 on the original 6–20 Borg scale.

2. RPE is considered a reliable indicator of exercise intensity and is particularly useful when a participant is unable to monitor their pulse or when HR response to exercise has been altered by medications **(Franklin et al, 2000).**

Calculating intensity: Owing to limitations in using VO2 calculations for prescribing intensity, the most common methods

60

of setting the intensity of exercise to improve or maintain cardiorespiratory fitness use HR and RPE **(Pollock et al,1998).**

Heart rate methods: HR is used as a guide to set exercise intensity because of the relatively linear relationship between HR and percentage of VO2max (%VO2max). It is best to measure HRmax during a progressive exercise test whenever possible since HRmax declines with age. HRmax can be estimated by using the following equation:

$$HRmax = 220 - age$$

This estimation has significant variance with a standard deviation of 10–12 beats per minute **(Franklin et al, 2000b) (Pollock et al, 1998).**

HRmax method: One of the oldest methods of setting the target HR range uses a straight percentage of the HRmax. Using 70–85% of an individual's HRmax approximates 55–75% VO2max and provides the stimulus needed to improve or maintain cardiorespiratory fitness **(Franklin et al, 2000) (Pollock et al, 1998).**

Example: If HRmax equals 180 bpm then target HR (70–85% HRmax) would range between 126–152 bpm.

61

Heart rate reserve method: The HR reserve (HRR) method is also known as the Karvonen method.

220-age = maximum HR

Reserve HR = maximum HR- resting HR.

Target HR = reserve HR × intensity % + resting HR

Using the HR method allows a more direct correlation between HR and % VO2 max **(Franklin et al., 2000) (Pollock et al., 1998).**

Rating of perceived exertion: Use of RPE is considered an adjunct to monitoring HR. It has proven to be a valuable aid in prescribing exercise for individuals who have difficulty with HR palpation, and in cases where the HR response to exercise may have been altered owing to a change in medication. The average RPE range associated with physiologic adaptation to exercise is 12–16 ("somewhat hard" to "hard") on the category Borg scale. One should suit the RPE to the individual on a specific mode of exercise and not expect an exact matching of the RPE to a %HRmax or %HRR. It should be used only as a guideline in setting the exercise intensity **(Franklin et al., 2000b) (Pollock et al., 1998).**

Finally, the appropriate exercise intensity is one that is safe and compatible with a long-term active lifestyle for that individual and achieves the desired outcome given the time constraints of the exercise session.

Duration

The ACSM recommends 20–60 min of continuous aerobic activity. However, deconditioned individuals may benefit from multiple, short-duration exercise sessions 10 min with frequent interspersed rest periods.

An inverse relationship exists between the intensity and duration of training. There may be greater musculoskeletal and cardiovascular risk with exercise performed at high intensities for short durations as compared with lower intensity exercise for a longer duration **(Franklin et al., 2000) (Pollock et al., 1998).**

Frequency

The ACSM recommends that aerobic exercise performed 3–5 days per week for most individuals. Less conditioned people may benefit from lower intensity, shorter duration exercise performed at higher frequencies per day and/or per week **(Franklin et al., 2000).**

Progression (Overload)

The rate of progression depends on health/fitness status , individual goals, and compliance rate. Frequency, intensity, and/or duration can be increased to provide overload. The goal for most healthy individuals is 30 min, 3–4 days per week at 85% HRR **(Franklin et al, 2000).**

Muscular Strength Training

Overload and specificity are precepts of resistance training. Overload occurs when a greater than normal physical demand is placed on muscles or muscle groups. Muscular strength and endurance are developed by increasing the resistance to movement or the frequency or duration of activity to levels above those normally experienced. A training intensity of approximately 40–60% of one repetition maximum (1 RM) appears to be sufficient for the development of muscular strength in most normally active individuals **(Franklin et al., 2000b) (Bryant and Peterson, 2001).**

Defining the terms "strength training" or "resistance training" may be a little more difficult than it seems at first glimpse. A number of variables such as; type of exercise, order of exercises, load or intensity, total volume of exercises and rest are obvious parameters that can be regulated in a training regimen **(Fleck and Kraemer, 2004).**

Specificity relates to the nature of changes (structural and functional, systemic and local) that occur in an individual as a result of training. These adaptations are specific and occur only in the overloaded muscle groups or muscles **(Durstine et al., 2001).**

The ACSM Provides the Following Guidelines for Resistance Training:

A 5–10-min warm-up period consisting of aerobic activity or a light set (50–75% of training weight) of the specific resistance exercise should precede the resistance exercise program. The goal is to develop total body strength and endurance in a time-efficient manner **(Bryant and Peterson, 2001).**

Mode

The prescription should include a minimum of 8 to 10 separate exercises that target major muscle groups (arms, shoulder, chest, abdomen, back, hips and legs). Free weights and weight machines are commonly used; however, springs, surgical or rubber tubing, and electronic devices are also used for resistance training **(Franklin et al., 2000).**

Intensity/Duration

Perform a minimum of one set of 8 to 12 repetition of each of the exercises to the point of volitional fatigue. Volitional fatigue refers to the inability to move a resistance through the appropriate range of motion with proper mechanical form. A set of 10 to 15 repetitions is recommended for developing muscular endurance and for those who are older or frailer **(Franklin et al., 2000).**

Frequency

Perform these exercises 2 to 3 days per week, usually with a day of rest in between **(Franklin et al., 2000b).**

Progression

Resistance may be increased when 12 repetitions can be completed with good technique **(Franklin et al., 2000b).**

Additional Recommendations

a. Perform every exercise through a full range of motion using proper technique and in a controlled manner including the lifting (concentric phase) and lowering (eccentric phase).

b. Maintain a normal breathing pattern and avoid breath holding (Valsalva).

c. Exercise with a partner when possible to provide feedback, assistance, and motivation **(Bryant and Peterson, 2001).**

Musculoskeletal Flexibility Training

Stretching Techniques

Static stretching:

Static stretching involves slowly stretching a muscle to the point of mild discomfort and then holding that position for an extended period of time (usually 10 to 30 s). It is effective, requires little time and the risk of injury is low. It is the most commonly recommended method.

Ballistic stretching:

Ballistic stretching uses the momentum created by repetitive bouncing movement to produce muscle stretch. This type of stretch can result in muscle soreness or injury and is generally not recommended **(Fredette, 2001).**

Proprioceptive neuromuscular facilitation (PNF):

Proprioceptive neuromuscular facilitation (PNF) involves a combination of alternating contraction and relaxation of both agonist and antagonist muscles through a designated series of motions. It is effective, but it is time consuming, requires a partner and may cause residual muscle soreness and has potential for injury if applied too vigorously **(Fredette, 2001).**

Flexibility exercises should be performed in a slow controlled manner with a gradual progression to greater ranges of motion. It is recommended that an active warm-up precede vigorous stretching exercises **(Franklin et al, 2000b; Fredette, 2001).**

Mode

A general stretching routine that exercises the major muscle and/or tendon groups using static or PNF techniques.

Intensity

Stretch the muscle to a position of mild discomfort.

68

Duration

10 to 30 sec. for static stretches and a 6 sec. contraction followed by a 10- 30 sec assisted stretch for PNF. Repeat the stretch 3–4 times.

Frequency

Minimum of 2 to 3 days per week **(Franklin et al, 2000; Fredette, 2001)**

General Components Of An Exercise Program

Once the exercise prescription has been formulated, it is integrated into a comprehensive physical conditioning program which consists of the following components:

1. Warm-up phase (10 min): Warm-up phase facilitates the transition form rest to exercise, stretches postural muscles, augments blood flow, and increases the metabolic rate from the resting level (1 MET) to the aerobic requirements for endurance training.

2. Endurance phase (20–60 min): Endurance phase develops cardiorespiratory fitness and includes 20 to 60 min of

continuous or intermittent (minimum of 10min bouts accumulated throughout the day)

3. Cooling down (5–10 min): This phase provides a period of gradual recovery from the endurance phase and includes exercises of diminishing intensities. It permits appropriate circulatory adjustments and return of the HR and BP to near resting values **(Wygand, 2001).**

While endurance training activities should be performed 3 to 5 days a week, complementary flexibility and resistance training may be undertaken at a slightly reduced frequency of 2 to 3 days a week. Flexibility training can be included as part of the warm-up or cool-down, or undertaken at a separate time.

Resistance training is often performed on alternate days when endurance training is not; however, both activities can be combined into the same workout **(Franklin et al., 2000b) (Wygand, 2001).**

Rate Of Progression

The recommended rate of progression in an exercise conditioning program depends on functional capacity, medical and health status, age, individual activity preferences and goals, and an individual's tolerance to the current level of training. For apparently healthy adults the endurance aspect of the exercise prescription has three stages of progression: initial, improvement, and maintenance **(Franklin et al., 2000b) (Wygand, 2001).**

Initial Conditioning

The initial stage should include light muscular endurance exercises and moderate level aerobic activities (40–60% of HRR), exercises that are compatible with minimal muscle soreness, discomfort and injury.

The duration of the exercise session during the initial stage may begin with approximately 15 to 20 min and progress to 30 min. It is recommended that individuals who are starting a moderate-intensity conditioning program should exercise 3 to 4 times per week **(Franklin et al., 2000) (Wygand, 2001).**

71

Improvement Stage

The goal of this stage of training is to provide a gradual increase in the overall exercise stimulus to allow for significant improvements in cardiorespiratory fitness. This stage typically lasts 4 to 5 months, during which intensity is progressively increased within the upper half of the target range of 50 to 85% of HR reserve. Duration is increased consistently every 2 to 3 weeks until participants are able to exercise at a moderate-to-vigorous intensity for 20 to 30 min continuously **(Wygand, 2001).**

Maintenance Stage

The goal of this stage of training is the long-term maintenance of cardiorespiratory fitness developed during the improvement stage. This stage of the exercise program usually begins after the first 5 or 6 months of training, but may begin at any time the participant has reached pre-established fitness goals. During this stage, the participant may no longer be interested in further increasing the conditioning stimulus. Further improvement may be minimal, but continuing the same workout routine enables individuals to maintain their fitness **(Franklin et al., 2000).**

72

Medical Clearance

Exercise training may not be appropriate for everyone .Patients whose adaptive reserves are severely limited by disease processes may be unable to adapt to or benefit from exercise. In this small subpopulation of people with severe or unstable cardiac, respiratory, metabolic, systemic, or musculoskeletal disease—exercise programming may be fatal, injurious, or simply not beneficial, depending on the clinical status and condition of the individual **(Franklin et al., 2000).**

Subjects and methods

This study was conducted on 30 apparently healthy volleyball players free from any medical or surgical illness, aging from 19-35 years and playing at Media Sporting Club and participating in the Egyptian volleyball league.

Exclusion criteria:

➤ Subjects suffering from other causes of increased serum cardiac troponin T (cTnT) such as sepsis, hypotension, supraventricular tachycardia, ingestion of sympathomimetic agents, cardiac contusion, pericarditis, cardiac transplantation, chemotherapy, congestive heart failure and chronic renal insufficiency.

➤ Subjects with known causes of pathological left ventricular hypertrophy such as hypertension, hypertrophic cardiomyopathy or positive family history of hypertrophic cardiomyopathy.

➤ Subjects taking any form of medication that affects diastolic function of the heart such as beta blockers, calcium channel blockers or steroids or any banned drugs

➢ Subjects who participate in any form of regular exercise during the off season period (2 months).

The study started at the beginning of the training cycle at the beginning of season 2008-2009 and season 2009-2010 after stoppage of training for 8 weeks and the players were subjected to the following:

1- Full medical history taking with emphasis on sport medicine history including:

- Full detailed history taking including name, age, gender, residence, occupation, marital status, and special habits of medical importance.

- Duration of sport playing, previous sport injury, onset of injury, mechanism of injury and methods of treatment.

2- Thorough clinical examination including:

a- General examination

Routine general examination was done with special emphasis on resting heart rate and resting blood pressure also anthropometric measures were done including height, weight and BMI where a scale was used to measure body weight (BW)

76

with an accuracy of ±100g. Subjects were weighted without shoes. Standing body height (BH) was measured with the use of a commercial stadiometer with the shoulders in relaxed position and arms hanging freely. Body mass index (BMI) was calculated as BW in kilograms (kg) divided by the square of the BH in meter (m2).

b-Local cardiac examination
Including inspection, palpation and auscultation.

3- 12 lead surface ECG .
Resting ECG was done to exclude any conduction abnormality of the heart.

4- Echocardiography

Echocardiographic and Doppler studies were performed with a Sonoline CD Siemens instrument equipped with a 2.5 MHz transducer. At rest, subjects were positioned at 30° left lateral position (fig 7) or in supine position (fig 8). An integrated M-mode and two-dimensional study was done to determine:

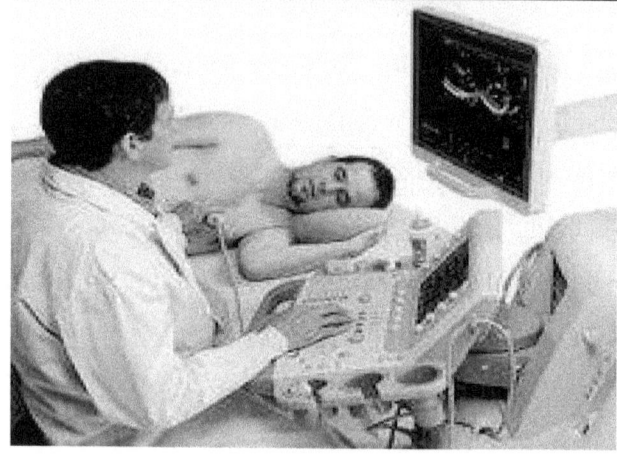

Fig 7 : Echocardiographic test in left lateral position. Quoted from http://radiologydegreeonline.net

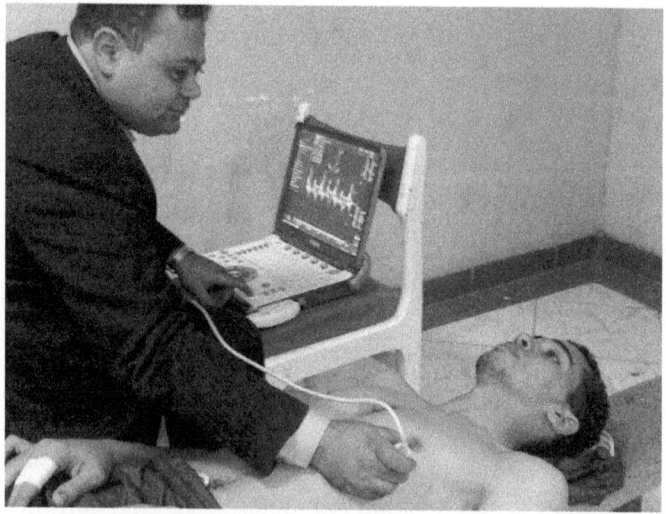

Fig 8: Echocardiography in supine position in our study.

A) Measures of cardiac structure include:

i-Left ventricular end diastolic dimension (LVEDD) (fig. 9), with normal values in men between 42 and 59 mm **(Lang et al., 2005).**

ii- Posterior wall thickness (PWT), and Interventricular septal thickness (IVST) (fig. 9), with normal values in men between 6 and 12 mm **(Barbier et al., 2006).**

iii -Left ventricular end systolic dimension (LVESD) (fig. 9) with normal values in men between 20 and 38 mm **(louise et al., 2005).**

iv- Left ventricular mass index (LVMI) was calculated as follows:

LVMI (gm/m²) = $\dfrac{0.0832 \times [(IVST + LVEED + PWT)3 - (LVESD)3] + 0.6}{BSA}$

with normal values in men between 55 and 116 gm/m² **(Spencer et al., 2005) (louise et al., 2005).**

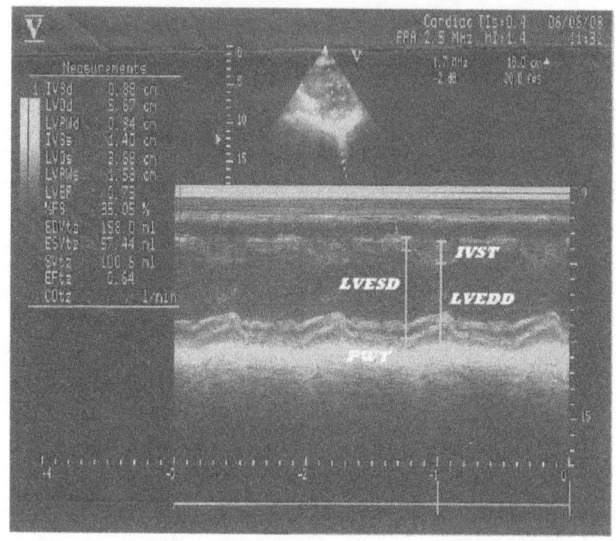

IVST: Interventricular septal thickness, LVEDD: Left ventricular end diastolic dimension, LVESD: Left ventricular end systolic dimension and PWT: Posterior wall thickness.

Fig 9: Echocardiography showing Cardiac chambers diameters and systolic function from our study.

B)Measures of systolic function include:

i-Stroke volume (SV) which is measured by subtracting end diastolic volume (EDV) from end systolic volume (ESV) with normal values in men more than 70 ml.

ii- Ejection fraction (EF) with normal values in men $\geq$ 55 %.

$$EF= \frac{stroke\ volume}{EDV}$$

iii- Fractional shortening (FS) with normal values in men between 25 and 43 % (Lang et al., 2005).

$$FS= \frac{LVEDD-LVESD}{LVEDD} \times 100$$

B) Measures of diastolic function :

i- Color M-mode Doppler flow propagation velocity (Vp) (figure 10), with normal values in men $\geq$ 45 cm/sec **(Moller et al., 2000).**

81

ii- Deceleration time (DT) (fig. 10,11) with normal values between 140 and 240 ms **(Moller et al., 2000).**

iii- E/A ratio was also calculated by determining peak E (early filling) and peak A (late atrial filling) (fig. 10,11) which is 1-2 in normal individuals **(gottdiener et al., 2004).**

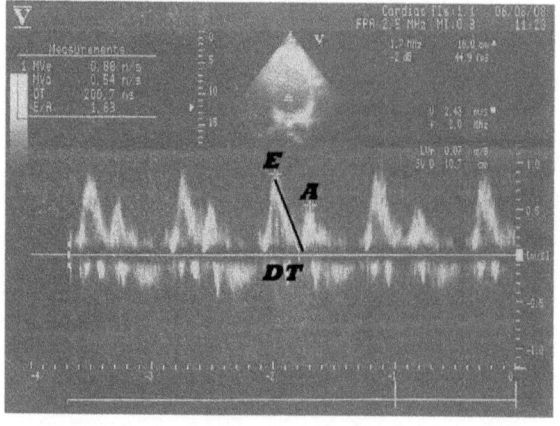

E: peak early filling, A: peak late atrial filling and DT: deceleration time.

Figure 10 : Echocardiography showing diastolic function from our study.

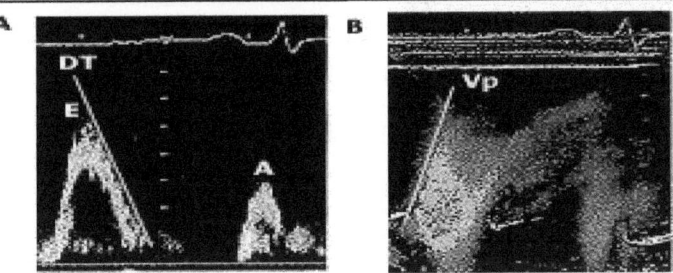

E: peak early filling, A: peak late atrial filling
DT: deceleration time and Vp: propagation
velocity.

.

Figure 11: Color M-mode Doppler showing diastolic function. Quoted from Moller et al., 2000.

5- Measuring serum cardiac troponin T (cTnT).

Five milliliters of venous blood were taken by sterile syringe in plastic tubes. Blood samples were centrifuged at 3000g for 5 minutes; sera were separated in clean tubes and stored in aliquots at -70oC until assayed.

Determination of serum cTnT was performed on the Elecsys 2010 system (Boehringer Mannheim) using the electrochemiluminiscence immunoassay (ECLIA). The minimum detection limit was 0.01 ng/ml; a level of >0.10 ng/ml was considered positive **(Stolear et al., 1999).**

The test is based on the sandwich principle. In the first incubation, using 15 µl of sample, a biotinylated monoclonal troponin T-specific antibody and a monoclonal troponin T-specific antibody labeled with a ruthenium complex react to form a sandwich complex. In the second incubation, after the addition of streptavidin-coated microparticles, the complex becomes bound to the solid phase via interaction of biotin and streptavidin. The reaction mixture is aspirated into the measuring cell where the microparticles are magnetically captured onto the surface of the electrode. Unbound substances are then removed with ProCell. Application of a voltage to the electrode then induces chemiluminiscent emission which is measured by a photomultipier **(Stolear et al., 1999).**

6- Measuring maximal O2 consumption of the muscles (Vo2 max)

VO2 max has been defined as the highest rate of oxygen consumption attainable during maximal or exhaustive exercise **(Wilmore and Costill 2005).**

In our study we measured the VO2 max by Zan 600 ergospirometry apparatus (fig. 12). The exercise test was performed on a Jaeger 6000 LE motor-driven treadmill, which was connected to the Zan 600 apparatus. The speed of the treadmill was 12 km/h. The slope of the treadmill was increased by 2.5% every 2 minutes. Concentration and volume of oxygen and carbon dioxide in the expired air were determined by special sensor at the connected mask (fig 13), the aerobic power refers to body mass related maximal oxygen uptake and measured as ml/kg/min (fig 14, 15, 16). Vo2 max values have a wide range and depends on the sex and age of the subject and the type of exercise practised as shown in table 2 and 3 **(Kneffel et al., 2007).**

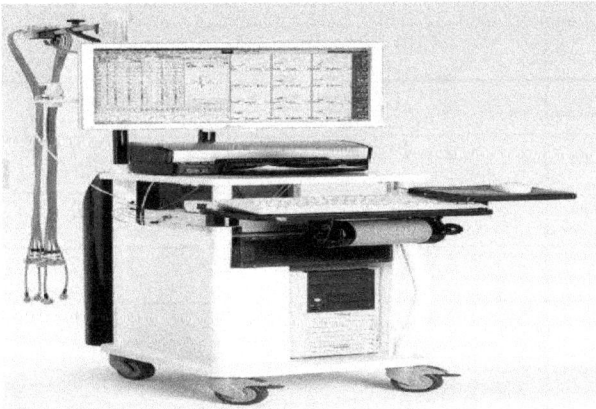

Figure 12: Zan 600 ergospirometer from the apparatus manual.

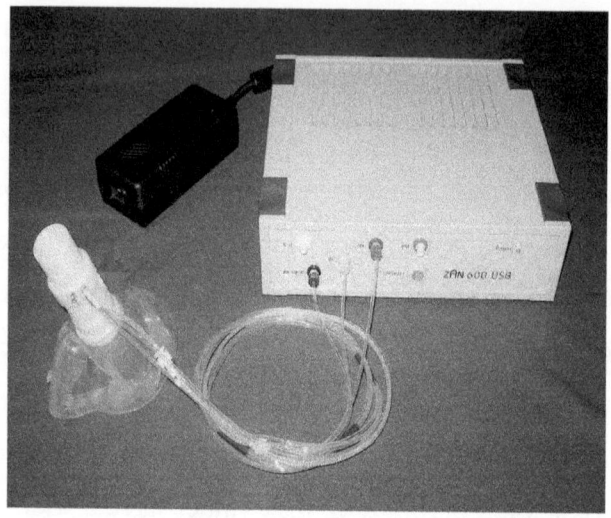

Figure 13: Zan 600 control unit with connected mask, ergo flow sensor and power supply.

Table 2: Normal Vo2 max values in ml/kg/min in non athletes.

Age	Male	Female
10-19	47-56	38-46
20-29	43-52	33-42
30-39	39-48	30-38
40-49	36-44	26-35
50-59	34-41	24-33
60-59	31-38	22-30

Quoted from Wilmore and Costill 2005.

Table 3 : Vo2 max in ml/kg/min in some athletes.

Sport	Age	Male	Female
Soccer	22-28	54-64	50-60
Basketball	18-30	40-60	43-60
Volleyball	18-28	NA	40-56
swimming	10-25	50-70	40-60
Weightlifting	20-30	38-52	NA
Cycling	18-26	31-38	22-30
Skiing	18-30	65-94	60-75
Wrestling	20-30	52-65	NA

Quoted from Wilmore and Costill 2005.

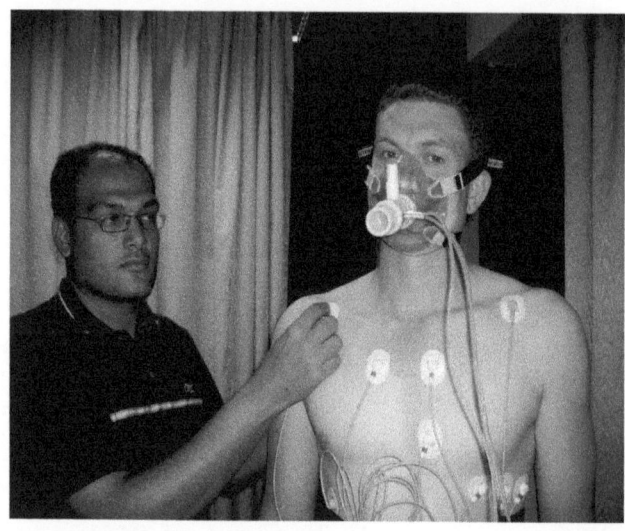

Figure 14: Applying ECG leads and the respiratory mask in our study.

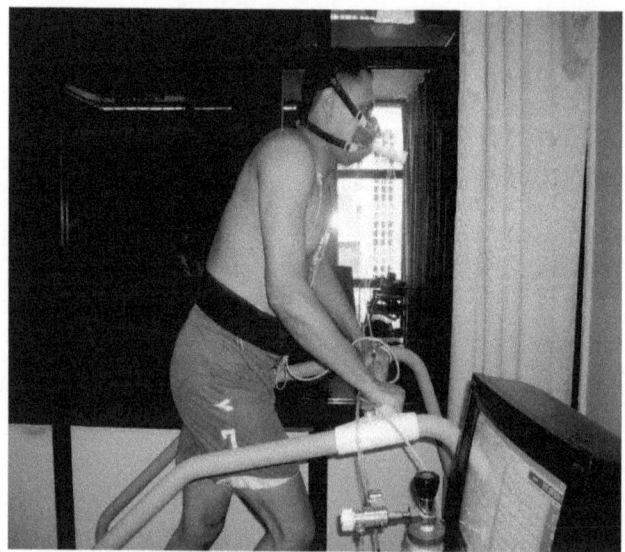

Figure 15: A player performing the test in our study.

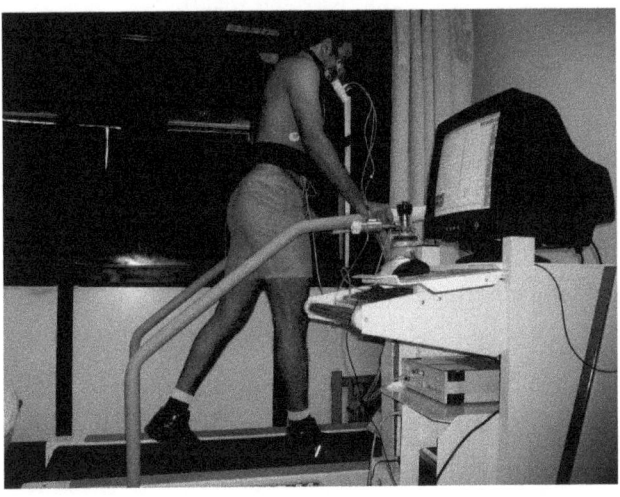

Figure 16: A player performing the test in our study where the Zan 600 was connected to the treadmill with the mask connected to the control unit.

ZAN Messgeräte GmbH
Schlimpfhofer Str. 14
D-97723 Oberthulba
Tel. 09736-8181-0, Fax. 09736-8181-20

Kareem, Ibrahim
ID-Nr: Karlbr200883
Comment:

193 cm, 85 kg, male *20.08.1983 =24Y
Test: 27.07.2008 / 10:01 h

Sport Test Report

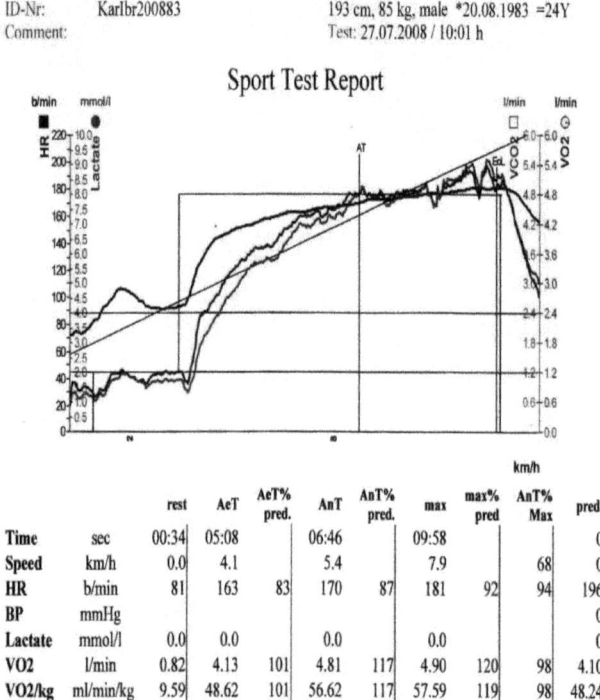

		rest	AeT	AeT% pred.	AnT	AnT% pred.	max	max% pred	AnT% Max	pred.
Time	sec	00:34	05:08		06:46		09:58			0
Speed	km/h	0.0	4.1		5.4		7.9		68	0
HR	b/min	81	163	83	170	87	181	92	94	196
BP	mmHg									0
Lactate	mmol/l	0.0	0.0		0.0		0.0			0
VO2	l/min	0.82	4.13	101	4.81	117	4.90	120	98	4.10
VO2/kg	ml/min/kg	9.59	48.62	101	56.62	117	57.59	119	98	48.24

AeT: aerobic training, AnT: anaerobic training, pred: predicted , HR: heart rate, BP: blood pressure.

Figure 17: Vo2 max report taken from one of our subjects showing Vo2 max equals 57.59.

90

The Training Program

The formulation of a program of exercise should begin with an identification of the person's goals. Would the person benefit most from increases in strength, increases in aerobic power, or a combination both **(Knuttgen 2007).**

The important considerations that then follow are the selection of the activity, the identification of the intensity of effort ,the identification of the repetitions and/or time involvement for each exercise session, and the weekly program **(Wilmore 2003).**

The training program was in the form of combined strengthening and endurance exercises with frequency of training 6 times/week for 12 weeks in the form of three days strengthening exercise alternating with another three days of endurance exercises, each training session was 45-60 minutes.

Endurance exercise program: (3 days/week, 45-60 minutes/day)

The factors to be considered are again the activity, the intensity, the duration of individual bouts, and the weekly program. To bring about changes in the circulatory system, the activity must necessarily involve a large portion of the person's skeletal muscle. Therefore, the activity could be chosen from walking, jogging, running, cycling, swimming, rowing, cross-country skiing, or on an exercise machine where these activities are simulated in our study we used running in field track around a soccer field this field track measures 400 meters.

The intensity should be sufficiently high to elicit a high percentage (50–80%) of the person's peak aerobic power (Vo2max) for the particular activity or 50–85% of reserve heart rate can be used, this target heart rate was calculated using Karvonen formula **(Karvonen et al., 1957), (Deuster and Keyser, 2005).**

220-age = maximum HR

Reserve HR = maximum HR- resting HR.

Target HR = reserve HR × intensity % + resting HR

For example if a player aged 30 years and his resting HR is 60 beat/min then his target HR was calculated as follows:

MHR = 220-30=180 b/min.

RHR = 180- 60 = 120 b/min.

Target HR = 120 × 0.5 + 60 = 120 b/min

120 × 0. 85 + 60 = 162 b/min

Then the heart rates for performance at these oxygen uptakes would be in the range of 120 to 162 beat /min, Although there are various systems for quantifying the person's perception of exertion, the simplest approach was to advise the player to exercise at an intensity that is perceived as physiologically challenging but, yet, can be carried on continuously or for the duration of the exercise period.

The total duration of the exercise period was between 45-60 minutes. The frequency was 3 times/week.

Each session starts with 10 minutes of running for warming up followed by 10 minutes of stretching exercises to all muscles of both lower limbs and each session ends by stretching exercises to the same muscles for 5 minutes. Stretching was Static stretching by assuming a stretch position and hold it for

93

30 seconds. There was no bouncing or rapid movement. And the player was instructed that he should feel mild pulling sensation, but no pain fig (18, 19, 20).

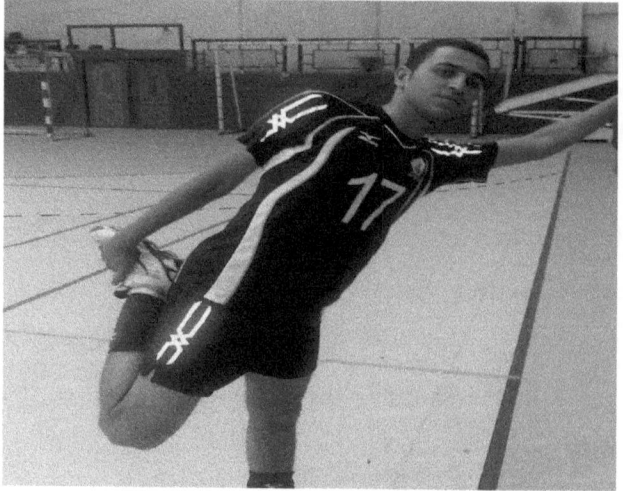

Figure 18 : A player performing static stretching to right quadriceps muscle taken from our study.

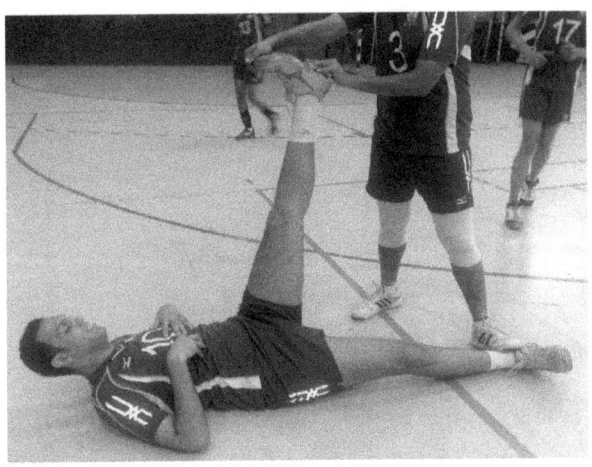

Figure 19: A player performing static stretching to left hamstring and calf muscles aided by a teammate taken from our study.

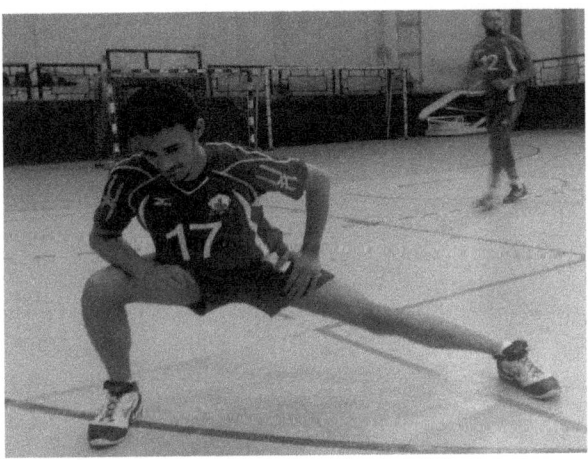

Figure 20: A player performing static stretching to left adductor group muscles taken from our study.

A- First month:

After the period of warming up and stretching the player started by running for 20 minutes and instructed that he must cover at least the desired number of laps with increasing gradually the number of these laps as shown below but if the player finished the desired laps before the end of the 20 minutes he should continue to run till the end of the time :

1st week...............10 laps

2nd week...............11 laps

3rd week...............12 laps

4th week...............13 laps

Each lap is 400 meters.

B- Second month:

After the period of warming up and stretching the player was instructed to do:

➢ Running for 4 minutes to cover at least 3 laps.

➢ Jogging for 1 minute.

➢ Rest for 2 minutes.

The sequence of running, jogging and rest was repeated 4 times.

C)Third month:

After the period of warming up and stretching this period is divided into 4 weeks as follows:

1st week:

> ➢ Sprinting 100 meters at the least time for 2 times.
> ➢ Rest for 5 minutes
> ➢ Running 20 minutes to cover at least 11 laps.

2nd week:

> ➢ Sprinting 100 meters at the least time 2 times.
> ➢ Sprinting 30 meters at the least time once.
> ➢ Rest for 5 minutes
> ➢ Running 20 minutes to cover 12 laps.

3rd week:

> ➢ Sprinting 100 meters at the least time 2 times.
> ➢ Sprinting 30 meters at the least time twice.
> ➢ Rest for 5 minutes.
> ➢ Running for 20 minutes to cover at least 13 laps.

4th week:

> ➢ Sprinting 100 meters at the least time 2 times.
> ➢ Sprinting 30 meters at the least times 3 times.
> ➢ Rest for 5 minutes.
> ➢ Running for 20 minutes to cover at least 14 laps.

Strengthening exercise program: (3 days/week, 45-60 min/day)

Strengthening exercise may be accomplished by utilizing free weights, exercise machines in which weights are incorporated, or exercise machines in which the opposing force (or resistance) is provided by other means (e.g., electronically). **(Knuttgen, 2007).** In our study we used both free weights and manual machines.

When training with weights, the magnitudes of increase in muscle strength and muscle endurance depend on the specific training parameters: repetitions, sets, volume, and intensity **(Deuster and Keyser, 2005).**

Repetition maximum: The amount of force a subject can lift a given number of repetitions defines as repetition maximum (RM). For example, 1RM is the maximal force a subject can lift with one repetition **(Knuttgen, 2007).**

Repetitions: Repetitions reflect the number of consecutive times a particular weight is lifted without a rest period. For examples, repetitions could be 5, 10, 12 or 25.

Sets: The number of sets represents how many times the repetitions are repeated after a rest period. For example, a training session could consist of three sets of 10 repetitions.

Volume: Volume equates to the total number of times a weight was lifted (Sets × Reps). For example, if the session was three sets of 12 repetitions, the volume would be 3 × 12 or 36 repetitions. Volume indicates how much work was done: the greater the volume, the greater the total work.

Intensity: Intensity reflects the actual resistance lifted, and is expressed as a percent of the maximum weight (1RM). For example if the 1RM for a particular exercise is 80 kg, then a weight of 40 kg would be a 50% and 60 kg a 75% intensity **(Campos et al., 2002).**

In our study we Started with the determination of the 1 repetition maximum (1RM) . 1 RM is identified for each group of muscles separately and was done only once at the beginning of the training program **(Knuttgen, 2007).**

The repetitions in the program were 10 for each exercise, the number of sets were 3 with one minute rest between each set, the volume of the prescribed exercise was 30 for each group of muscles exercised (10 repetitions × 3 sets) and the intensity was as follows:

We Started with 50 % of 1RM for the first 4 weeks then increase to 60-70% of 1 RM for another 4 weeks then shifted to 80-90% of 1RM for the last 4 weeks. For each training session the player performs 3 sets of exercises for each group of muscles each set formed of 10 repetitions. The rest periods were 1 minute between each set and 1 minute between each group of muscles.

Each training session started with a period of warming up formed of running for 10 minutes and 5-10 minutes of stretching to the exercised muscles, the stretching was Static stretching by assuming a stretch position and hold it for 30 seconds. There was no bouncing or rapid movement. And the player was instructed that he should feel mild pulling sensation, but no pain.

The group of muscles included in this training program were:

Flexors, extensors, abductors and adductors of the shoulder (fig. 21 and 22).

Flexors and extensors of the elbow (figure 23 and 24).

Flexors and extensors of the wrist (figure 25).

Flexors and extensors of the knee (figure 26).

Adductors and abductors of the hip (figure 27).

Planter flexors and dorsiflexors of the ankle .

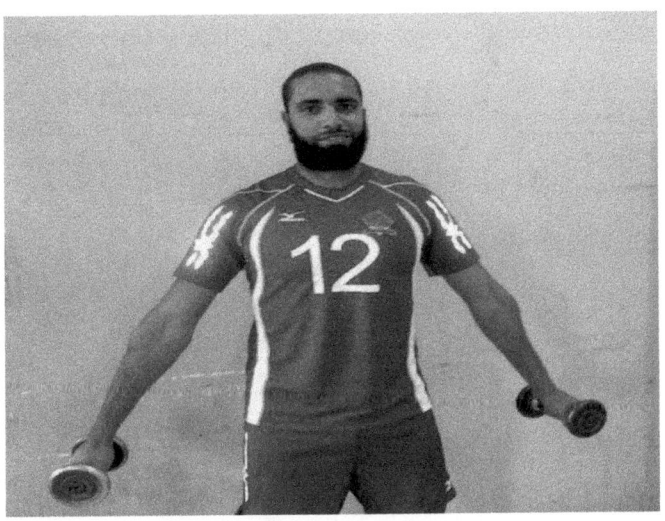

Figure 21: Strengthening exercise program for shoulder abductors muscle taken from our study

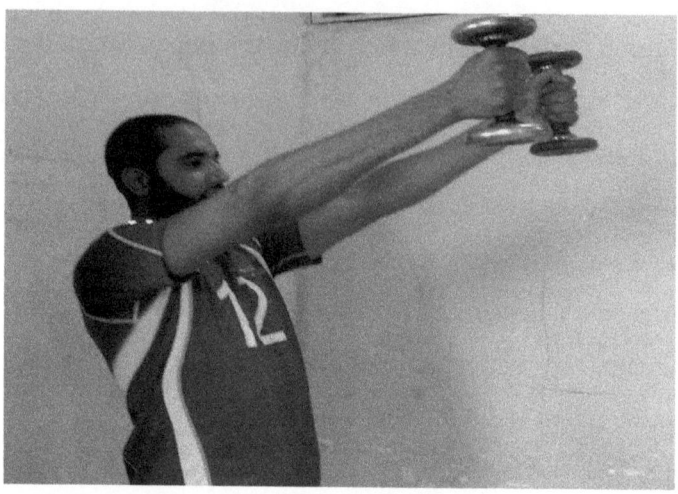

Figure 22: Strengthening exercise program for shoulder flexors muscle taken from our study

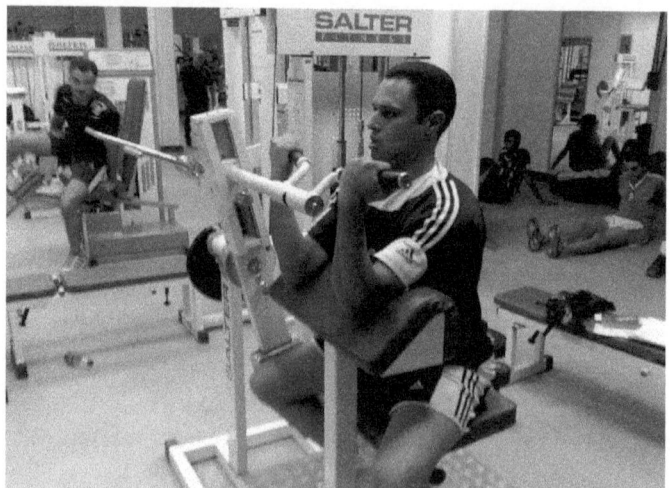

Figure 23: Strengthening exercise program for the biceps brachii muscle taken from our study.

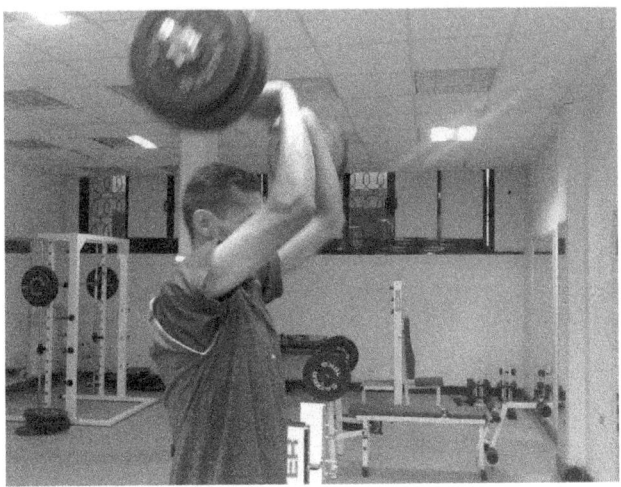

Figure 24: Strengthening exercise program for the triceps muscle taken from our study.

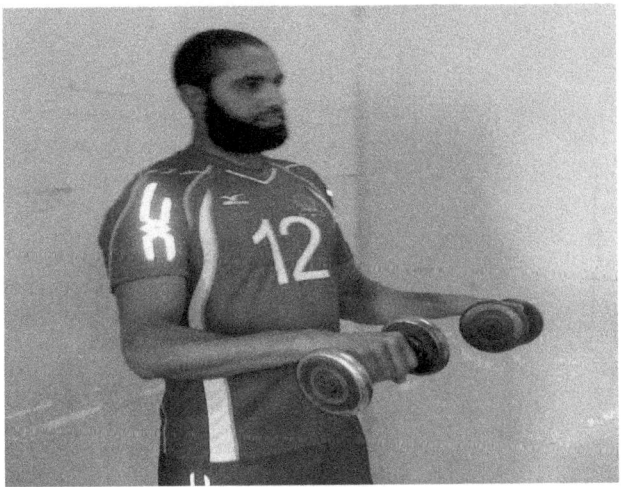

Figure 25: Strengthening exercise program for wrist extensors taken from our study.

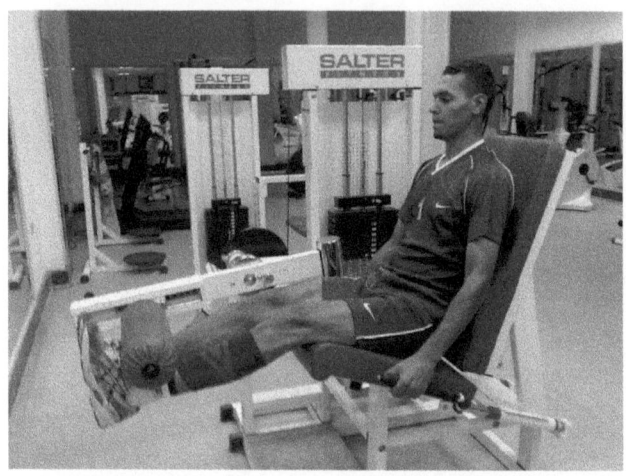

Figure 26: Strengthening exercise program for the quadriceps muscle taken from our study.

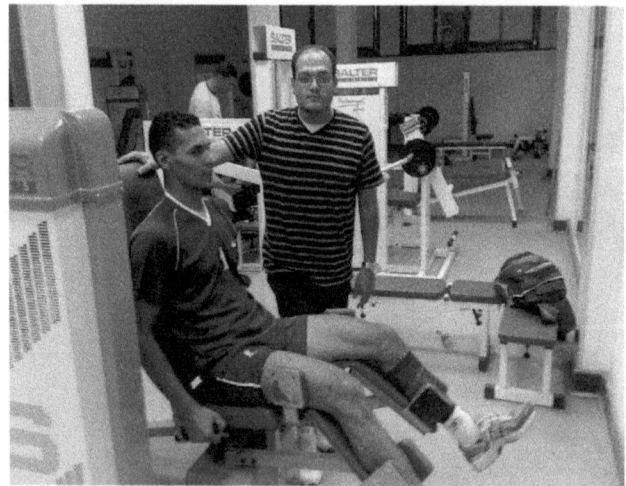

Figure 27: Strengthening exercise program for the adductors and abductors of the hip taken from our study.

Follow up

After 12 weeks of the combined strengthening and endurance training we repeated the following:

➢ Echocardiography which was done by the same sonographer.

➢ Serum cardiac troponin T (cTnT) using the same technique

➢ Maximal oxygen consumption (Vo2 Max) on the same device.

Data Management and Analysis:

The collected data will be revised, coded, tabulated and introduced to a PC using Statistical package for Social Science (SPSS 15.0.1 for windows; SPSS Inc, Chicago, IL, 2001). Data will be presented and suitable analysis will be done according to the type of data obtained for each parameter.

i-   Descriptive statistics:

Mean, Standard deviation (± SD), Minimum and maximum values (range) for numerical data.

ii- Analytical statistics:

1.Paired t-test will be used to assess the statistical significance of the difference between two means measured twice for the same study group.

2. Correlation analysis (using Pearson's method): To assess the strength of association between two quantitative variables. The correlation coefficient denoted symbolically "r" defines the strength and direction of the linear relationship between two variables.

106

Results

This study was conducted on 30 apparently healthy volleyball male players free from any medical or surgical illness, aging from 20-35 years and playing at Media Sporting Club and participating in the Egyptian volleyball league.

Demographic data:

The players were all males, their age ranged from 20 to 35 years with a mean of 26.27 ± 4.258. Their weight ranged from 64 to 102 kg with a mean of 85.20 ± 9.83, while their height ranged from 170 to 202 cm with a mean of 187.6 ± 7.27 and their BMI ranged from 19 to 28 Kg/m² with a mean of 24.31 ± 1.79 Kg/m² as shown in table 4.

Table 4: demographic data

	Minimum	Maximum	Mean ± SD
Age (years)	20	35	26.27 ± 4.258
Weight (kg)	64	102	85.20 ± 9.831
Height (cm)	170	202	187.6 ± 7.271
BMI (Kg/m²)	19	28	24.31 ± 1.79

BMI: body mass index

Vital data:

Their systolic blood pressure ranged from 100 to 130 mmHg with a mean of 116.17 ± 7.27 while their diastolic blood pressure ranged from 70 to 90 mmHg with a mean of 77 ± 6.77 and their resting heart rate ranged from 60 to 96 beat/min with a mean of 76.63 ± 8.04 this is shown in table 5.

Table 5: Vital data

	Minimum	Maximum	Mean ± SD
Systolic BP (mmHg)	100	130	116.17 ± 7.273
Diastolic BP (mmHg)	70	90	77.00 ± 6.772
Resting HR (beat/min)	60	96	76.63 ± 8.045

Description of echocardiographic cardiac structure

As regard cardiac structure the left ventricular end diastolic dimension (LVEDD) ranged from 47 to 58 mm with a mean of 53.7 ± 3.4. Left ventricular end systolic dimension (LVESD) ranged from 26 to 40 mm with a mean of 33.8 ± 3.7, while the interventricular septal thickness(IVST) ranged from 8 to 11.4 mm with a mean of 9.8 ± 0.9. Posterior wall thickness (PWT) ranged from 9 to 12 mm with a mean of 9.9 ± 0.8 and left ventricular mass index(LVMI) ranged from 69.1 to 139.3 gm/m^2 with a mean of 97.3 ± 15.5. All these values of cardiac structure are within normal range for the same age and sex group except LVESD which may be considered above normal in 3 players but some authors reported that LVESD could reach up to 40 mm in endurance athletes **(Thomson and Etes, 2007)**. Also LVMI was higher than normal in 3 players.

LVMI reported to reach up to 141 gm/m^2 in endurance athletes with eccentric left ventricular hypertrophy and up to 155 gm/m^2 in athletes with concentric left ventricular hypertrophy **(Mayet et al., 2002)** .This is shown in table 6.

Table 6: Description of echocardiographic cardiac structure.

	Minimum	Maximum	Mean ± SD
LVEDD (mm)	47.0	58.0	53.7 ± 3.4
LVESD (mm)	26.0	40.0	33.8 ± 3.7
IVST (mm)	8.0	11.4	9.8 ± 0.9
PWT (mm)	9.0	12.0	9.9 ± 0.8
LVMI (gm/m²)	69.1	139.3	97.3 ± 15.5

LVEDD: left ventricular end diastolic dimension, IVS : interventricular septal thickness, PW: posterior wall thickness, LVMI : left ventricular mass index , LVESD : left ventricular end systolic dimension.

Description of echocardiographic cardiac Systolic function

On measuring systolic function the stroke volume (SV) ranged from 78 to 158 ml with a mean of 116.6 ± 20.9, while the fraction (EF) ranged from 58 % to 80 % with a mean of 65.7 ± 5.7 and the fractional shortening (FS) ranged from 30.7 % to 53.5 % with a mean of 37 ± 4.9. All these values of systolic function are within normal range for the same age and sex group

except one player with FS equals 53.5 % which is above normal
as shown in table 7.

Table 7: Echocardiographic Systolic function

	Minimum	Maximum	Mean ± SD
SV (ml)	78	158	116.6 ± 20.9
EF (%)	58	80	65.7 ± 5.7
FS (%)	30.7	53.5	37.0 ± 4.9

SV: stroke volume, FS : fractional shortening, EF:
ejection fraction

Description of Echocardiographic cardiac Diastolic function.

As for the diastolic function the propagation velocity (Vp)
ranged from 46 to 92 cm/sec with a mean of 64.1 ± 10.44. These
values are within normal range for athletes in the same age and
sex. Deceleration time (DT) ranged from 111 to 242 msec with a
mean of 180.8 ± 34.38 these values are within normal range
except for 2 players where DT values were < 140 msec and this
may be pseudonormal left ventricular filling pattern and is
differentiated from restrictive diastolic dysfunction by Vp
which is > 45 cm/sec according to **Moller et al., 2000.**

E/A ratio ranged from 1 to 2.6 with a mean of 1.64 ± 0.39. These values of E/A ratio were within normal range except for 5 players where E/A were > 2 and this could be considered normal in athletes according to **Green et al., 2006.** This is shown in table 8.

Table 8 : Echocardiographic cardiac Diastolic function.

	Minimum	Maximum	Mean ± SD
Vp (cm/sec)	46.0	92.0	64.10 ± 10.44
DT (msec)	111.0	242.0	180.87 ±34.38
E/A ratio	1.0	2.6	1.64 ± 0.39

E/A : peak e/ peak a, DT: deceleration time, Vp: propagation velocity

Serum cardiac troponin T

On measuring serum cardiac Troponin T which is a highly sensitive and specific marker of acute myocardial injury it ranged from 0.02 to 0.08 ng/ml with a mean of 0.06 ± 0.02 as shown in table 9.

Table 9 : Serum cardiac troponin T

	Minimum	Maximum	Mean ± SD
Serum Troponin (ng/ml)	0.02	0.08	0.06 ± 0.02

Maximal O2 consumption of the muscles (Vo2 max)

Measuring Vo2 max is an indicator of the endurance capacity of athletes. On measuring Vo2 max in our study it ranged from 31.4 to 58.7 ml/min/kg with a mean of 50.76 ± 6.91. These results were within expected values for this group of players as shown in table 10.

Table 10 : Maximal O2 consumption of the muscles (Vo2 max)

	Minimum	Maximum	Mean ± SD
Vo2 max (ml/min/kg)	31.4	58.7	50.76 ± 6.91

A training program was prescribed to be performed by the players in the form of combined strengthening and endurance exercises with frequency of training 6 times/week for 12 weeks in the form of three days strengthening exercise alternating with another three days of endurance exercises, each training session was 45-60 minutes.

Description of echocardiographic cardiac structure after training

As regard echocardiographic cardiac structure after

training LVEDD ranged from 47 to 58 mm with a mean of 52.35± 3.2, while LVESD ranged from 29 to 39 mm with a mean of 34.15 ± 2.28. IVST ranged from 9 to 13 mm with a mean of 10.57 ± 0.73, while PWT ranged from 9 to 11 mm with a mean of 10.47 ± 0.63 and LVMI ranged from 76.9 to 124.8 gm/m² with a mean of 100.43 ± 12.12 as shown in table 11.

Table 11: Description of echocardiographic cardiac structure after training.

	Minimum	Maximum	Mean ± SD
LVEDD (mm)	47.0	58.0	52.35 ± 3.20
LVESD (mm)	29.0	39.0	34.15 ± 2.28
IVST (mm)	9.0	13.0	10.57 ± 0.73
PWT (mm)	9.0	11.0	10.47 ± 0.63
LVMI (gm/m²)	76.9	124.8	100.43 ± 12.12

LVEDD: left ventricular end diastolic dimension, IVS : interventricular septal thickness, PW: posterior wall thickness, LVMI : left ventricular mass index , LVESD : left ventricular end systolic dimension.

114

Description of echocardiographic cardiac Systolic function after training.

On measuring systolic function after training SV ranged from 65 to 140 ml with a mean of 104.2 ± 22.33, while EF ranged from 55% to 70 % with a mean of 63.1 ± 4.64 and FS ranged from 27.6% to 40.8 % with a mean of 34.63 ± 3.67 as shown in table 12.

Table 12 : Description of echocardiographic cardiac Systolic function after training.

	Minimum	Maximum	Mean ± SD
SV (ml)	65	140	104.2 ± 22.33
EF (%)	55	70	63.1 ± 4.64
FS (%)	27.6	40.8	34.63 ± 3.67

SV: stroke volume, FS : fractional shortening, EF: ejection fraction

Description of Echocardiographic cardiac Diastolic function. after training.

As for the diastolic function the Vp ranged from 55 to 105 cm/sec with a mean of 84.17 ± 12.29, while DT ranged from 89 to 235 msec with a mean of 171.37 ± 41.01 and E/A ratio ranged from 1.2 to 2 with a mean of 1.56 ± 0.24 this is shown in table 13.

Table 13: Description of Echocardiographic cardiac Diastolic function after training.

	Minimum	Maximum	Mean ± SD
Vp (cm/sec)	55	105	84.17 ± 12.29
DT (msec)	89	235	171.37 ±41.01
E/A ratio	1.2	2	1.56 ± 0.24

E/A: peak e/ peak a, DT: deceleration time, Vp: propagation velocity

Serum cardiac troponin T after training.

On measuring serum cardiac Toponin T it ranged from 0.02 to 0.09 ng/ml with a mean of 0.06 ± 0.02 as shown in table 14.

Table 14: Serum cardiac troponin T after training.

	Minimum	**Maximum**	**Mean ± SD**
Serum troponin T (ng/ml)	0.02	0.09	0.06 ± 0.02

Maximal O2 consumption of the muscles (Vo2 max) after training

On measuring Vo2 max after training it ranged from 40.3 to 67.1 ml/min/kg with a mean of 56.47 ± 7.25 as shown in table 15.

116

Table 15 : Maximal O2 consumption of the muscles (Vo2 max) after training.

	Minimum	Maximum	Mean ± SD
Vo2 max (ml/min/kg)	40.3	67.1	56.47 ± 7.25

Comparison between echocardiographic cardiac structure before and after training

There were highly significant differences as regard IVS and PWT before and after the training program where t = -3.889 and -3.798 respectively and p < 0.005 for both variants.

And there was significant difference in LVEDD before and after training where t = 2.546 and p< 0.05, while there were no significant differences in LVMI and LVESD before and after training where t = -1.212 and -0.528 respectively and p > 0.05 as shown in table 16 and figure 28.

Table 16: Comparison between echocardiographic cardiac structure before and after training.

	Mean ± SD	t	P	Sig
IVST(Pre)	9.78 ± 0.881	-3.889	0.001	HS
IVST (Post)	10.57 ± 0.728			
PWT (Pre)	9.90 ± 0.845	-3.798	0.001	HS
PWT (Post)	10.47 ± 0.629			
LVEDD (Pre)	53.7 ± 3.375	2.546	0.016	S
LVEDD (Post)	52.35 ± 3.203			
LVMI (Pre)	97.34 ± 15.48	-1.212	0.235	NS
LVMI (Post)	100.425 ± 12.11			
LVESD (Pre)	33.83 ± 3.677	-0.528	0.602	NS
LVESD (Post)	34.15 ± 2.279			

LVEDD: left ventricular end diastolic dimension, IVST : interventricular septal thickness, PWT: posterior wall thickness, LVMI : left ventricular mass index , LVESD : left ventricular end systolic dimension

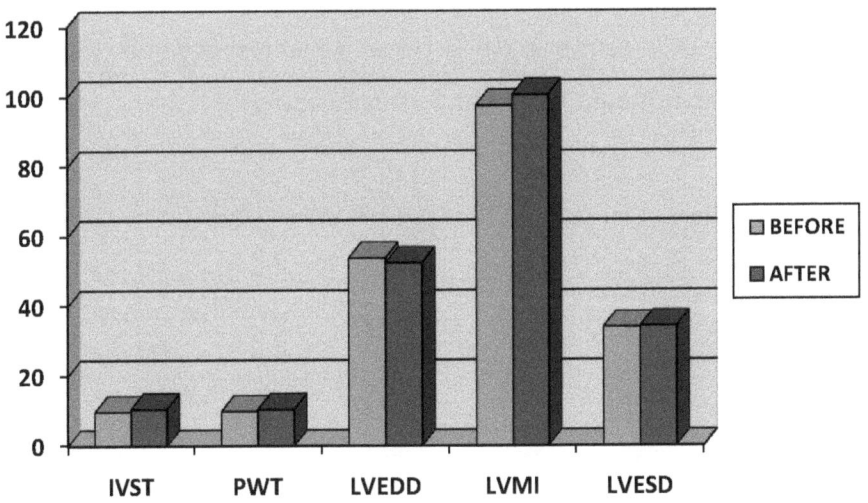

Figure 28: Highly significant difference in interventricular septal thickness (IVST), posterior wall thickness (PWT). And significant difference in left ventricular end diastolic dimension (LVEDD). While no significant difference in left ventricular mass index (LVMI) and left ventricular end systolic dimension (LVESD).

Comparison between echocardiographic cardiac systolic function before and after training.

There was highly significant difference in SV before and after training program where t = 3.668 and p< 0.005 . And there were significant differences in FS and EF before and after training where t = 2.714 and 2.350 respectively and p<0.05 as shown in Table 17 and figure 29.

119

Table 17: Comparison between echocardiographic cardiac systolic function before and after training.

	Mean ± SD	t	P	Sig
SV (Pre)	116.63 ± 20.908	3.668	0.001	HS
SV (Post)	104.20 ± 22.33			
FS (Pre)	37.017 ± 4.86	2.714	0.011	S
FS (Post)	34.633 ± 3.66			
EF (Pre)	65.70 ± 5.706	2.350	0.026	S
EF (Post)	63.10 ± 4.641			

SV: stroke volume, FS : fractional shortening, EF: ejection fraction

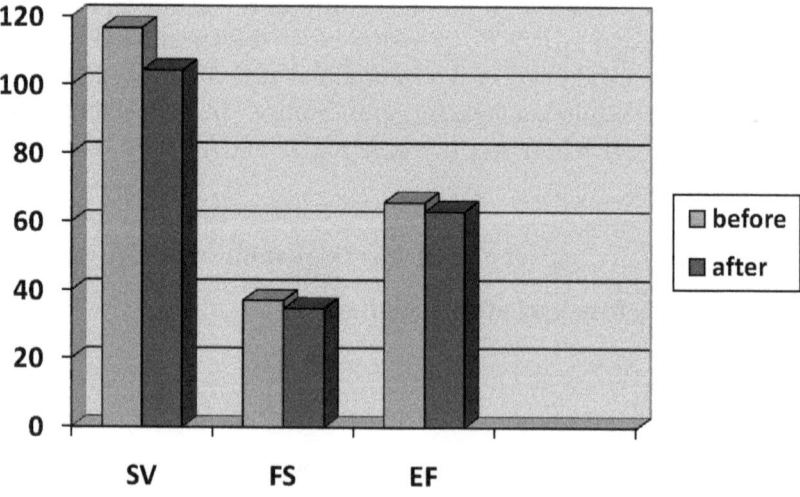

Figure 29: Highly significant difference in stroke volume (SV), and significant difference in fractional shortening (FS) and ejection fraction (EF) before and after training.

Comparison between echocardiographic cardiac Diastolic function before and after training

There was highly significant difference as regard Vp before and training program where t= -9.186 and p< 0.005. On the other hand there were no significant differences in E/A ratio and DT before and after training where t = 1.144 and 1.054 respectively and p > 0.05 as shown in table 18 and figure 30.

Table 18: Comparison between echocardiographic cardiac Diastolic function before and after training.

	Mean ± SD	t	P	Sig
Vp (Pre)	64.10 ± 10.443	-9.186	0.0001	HS
Vp (Post)	84.17 ± 12.287			
E/A(Pre)	1.6447 ± 0.392	1.144	0.262	NS
E/A(Post)	1.5590 ± 0.238			
DT (Pre)	180.87 ± 34.37	1.054	0.301	NS
DT (Post)	171.37 ± 41.01			

E/A : peak e/ peak a, DT: deceleration time, Vp: propagation velocity

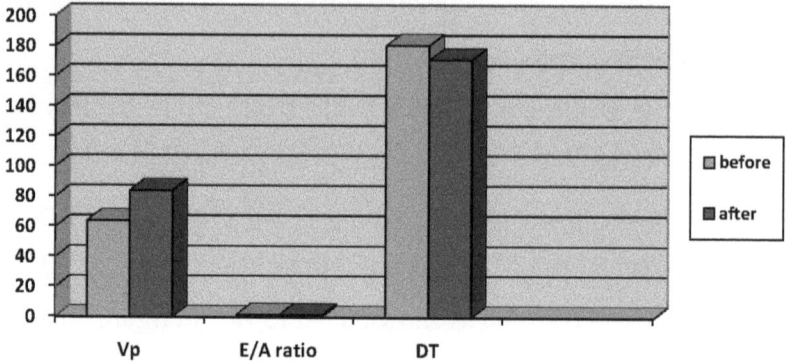

Figure 30: Highly significant difference in propagation velocity (Vp), and no significant differences in E/A ratio and deceleration time (DT) before and after training.

Comparison between serum cardiac troponin T before and after training program.

There was no significant differences in serum cardiac troponin T before and after training where t = -0.733 and p> 0.05 as shown in table 19 and figure 31.

Table 19: Comparison between serum troponin level before and after training.

	Mean	t	P	Sig
S.Troponin(pre)	0.0617 ± 0.0151			
		-0.733	0.470	NS
S.Troponin(post)	0.0637 ± 0.0154			

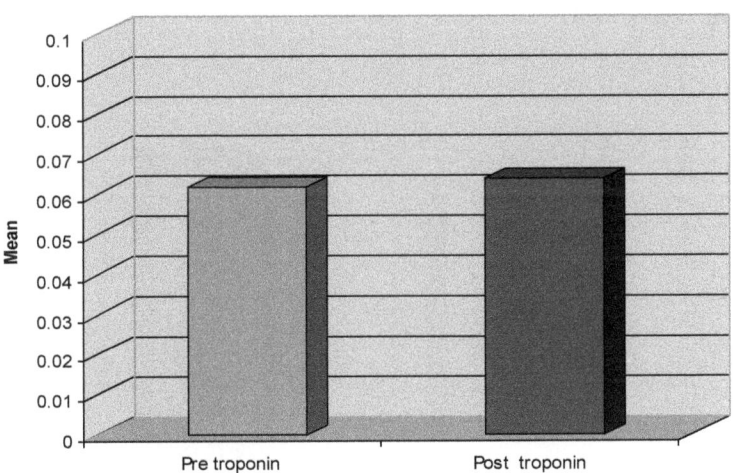

Figure 31 : No significant difference Between Serum cardiac Troponin T before and after training.

Comparison between Maximal O2 consumption of the muscles (Vo2 max) before and after training

On measuring Vo2 max, there was highly significant

difference as regard Vo2 max before and after training with
t= -12.72 and p< 0.005 as shown in table 20 and figure 32.

**Table 20: Comparison between Maximal O2 consumption of
the muscles (Vo2 max) before and after training.**

	Mean ± SD	t	P	Sig
Vo2 max (pre)	50.76 ± 6.90	-12.72	0.0001	HS
Vo2 max(post)	56.46 ± 7.24			

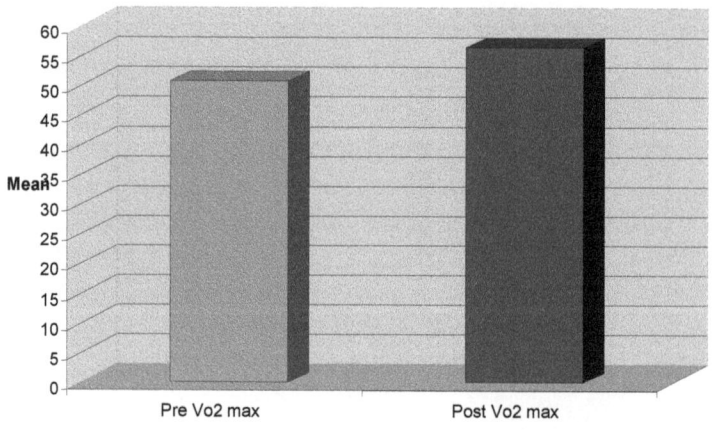

Figure 32 : Highly significant difference in Vo2 max before and
after training.

Statistical Correlations

Correlations between age and (diastolic function and Vo2 max before training:

Correlation studies showed a positive correlation between age and propagation velocity (Vp) before training as r= 0.486 and p< 0.05.this shown in fig (33). While there were no significant correlation between age and E/A, DT and Vo2 max before training.

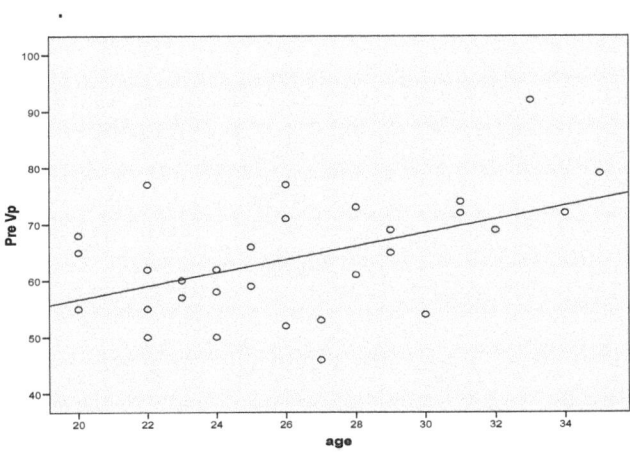

Figure 33: Correlation between age and propagation velocity (Vp) before training,

Correlations between BMI and (diastolic function and Vo2 max before training:

Correlation studies showed a positive correlation between body mass index (BMI) and deceleration time (DT) before training as r= 0.363 and p<0.05 this shown in fig (34). And there was significant negative correlation between BMI and Vo2 max before training as r= -0.406 and p< 0.05. as shown in fig. (35) While there were no significant correlation between BMI and E/A ratio and propagation velocity (Vp) before training.

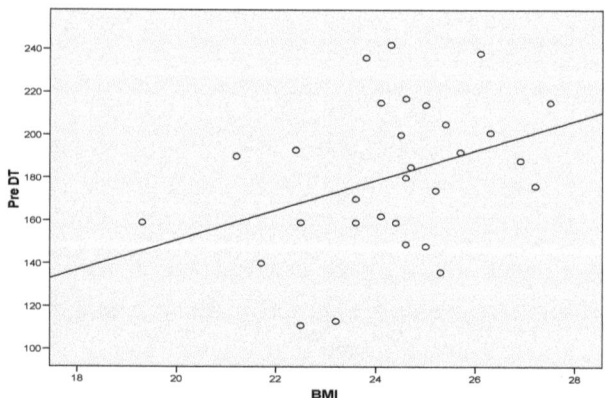

Figure 34 : Correlation between BMI and deceleration time (DT) before training.

126

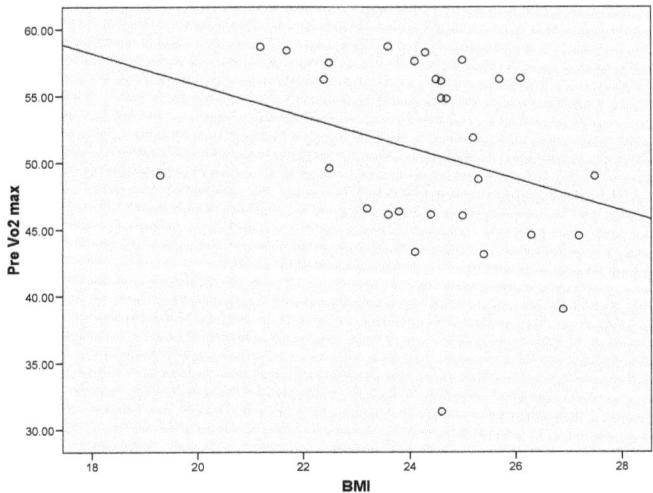

Figure 35 : Correlation between BMI and Vo2 max before training.

Correlations between VO2 max and diastolic function before training:

Correlation studies showed a positive correlation between Vo2 max and Vp before training as r=0.413, and P< 0.05. This is shown in figure (36). While there were no significant correlation between Vo2 max and E/A ratio and DT before training.

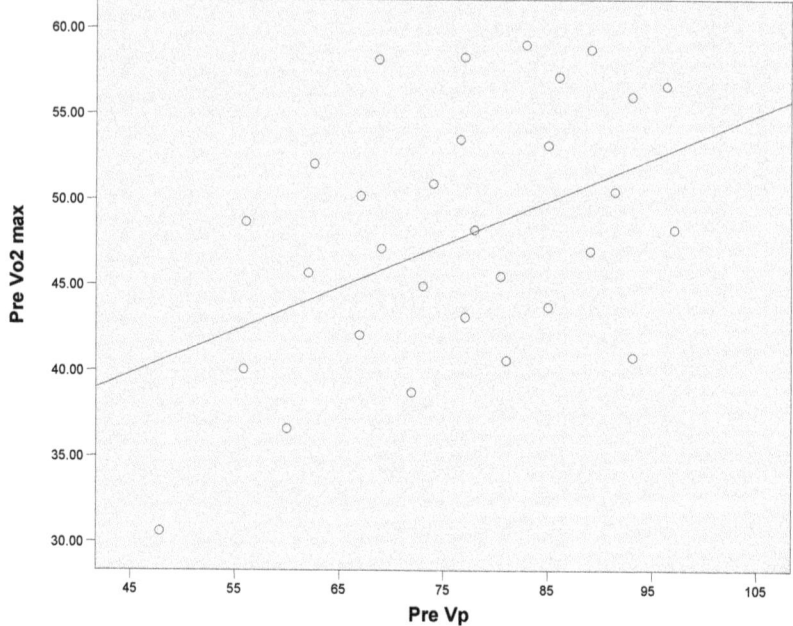

Figure 36: Correlation between Vo2 max and Vp before training.

Correlations between VO2 max and diastolic function after training:

There were significant positive correlation between Vo2 max and E/A ratio and Vp and after training as r= 0.325 and 0.318 respectivly with p < 0.05 for both correlations as shown in figures (37) and (38). While there was no significant correlation between   Vo2 max and DT max after training.

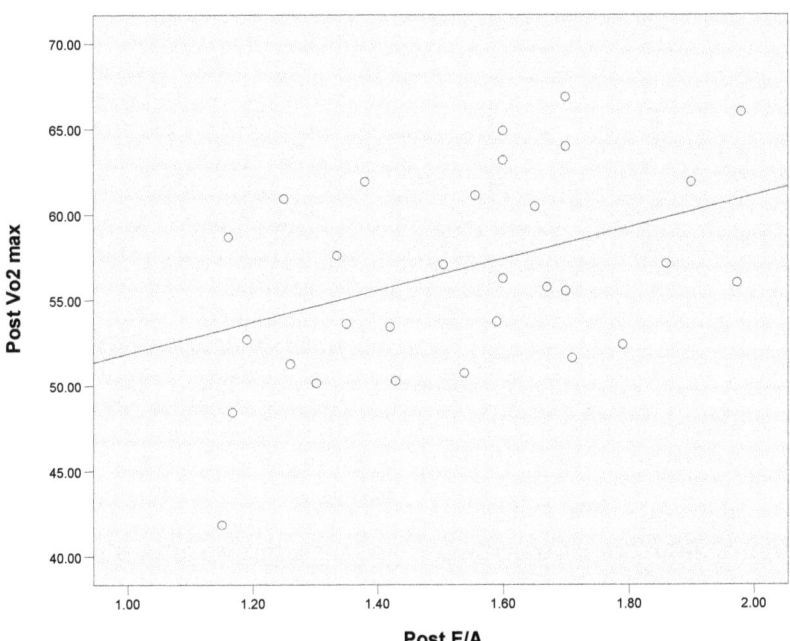

Figure 37: Correlation betweenVo2max and E/A ratio after training.

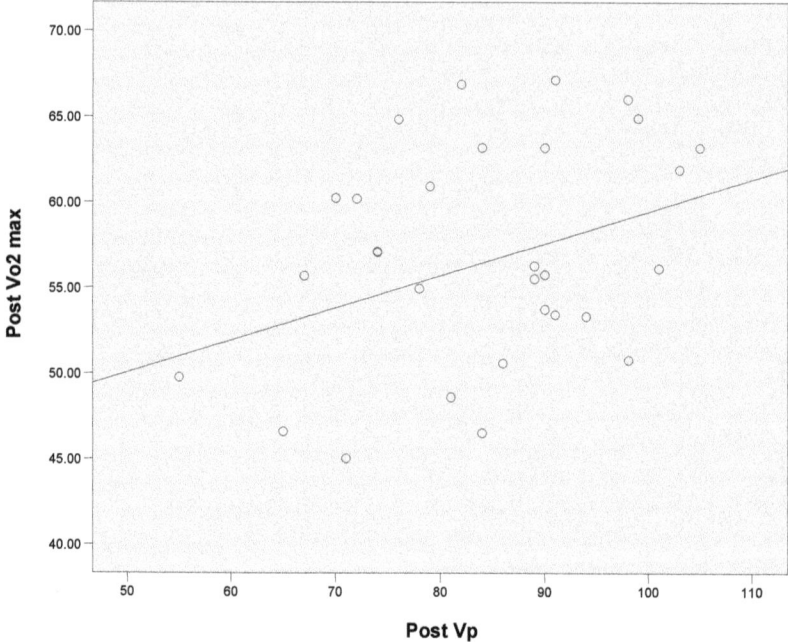

Figure 38: Correlation between Vo2 max and Vp after training.

Correlation between serum cardiac troponin T and diastolic function before training.

There were no significant correlations between serum cardiac troponin T and E/A ratio, DT and Vp before training with $r = 0.109$, 0.049 and 0.224 respectively and $p > 0.05$.

Correlations between serum cardiac troponin T and diastolic function after training.

There was highly significant positive correlation between serum cardiac troponin T and DT as r = 0.572 and p < 0.001as shown in figure 39. While there were no significant correlations between serum cardiac troponin T and E/A ratio and Vp as r = -0.29 and 0.171 respectively with p > 0.05.

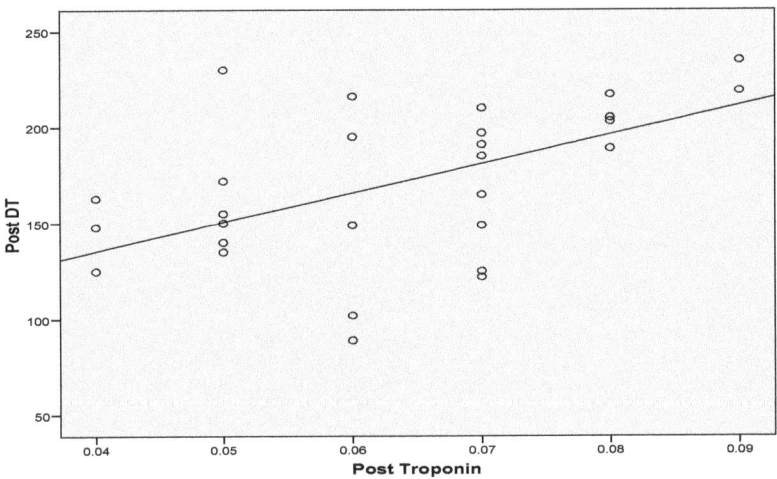

Figure 39 : Correlation between serum cardiac troponin T and DT after training.

131

Correlation between change in VO2 max and change in Vp .

There was significant positive correlation between change in Vo2 max and change in Vp as r = 0.351 and p < 0.05 as shown in figure 40.

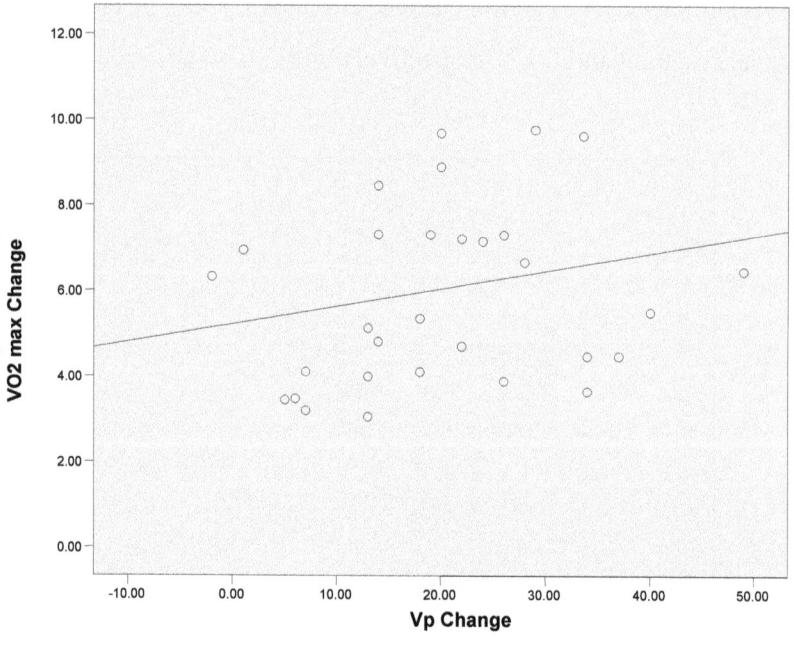

Figure 40: Correlation between change in VO2 max and change in Vp.

Correlation between change in VO2 max and change in E/A ratio:

There was significant positive correlation between changes in Vo2 max and changes in E/A ratio as r = 0.372 and p < 0.05 as shown in figure 41.

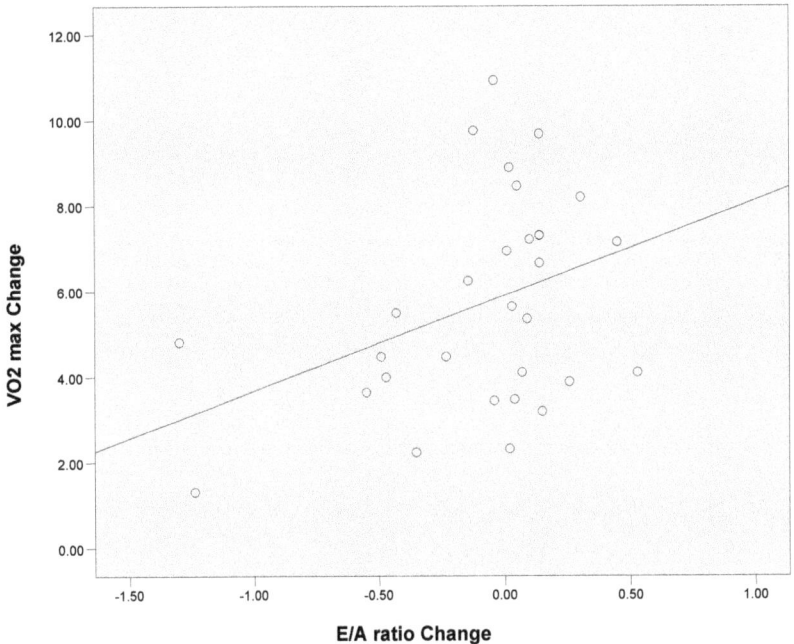

Figure 41: Correlations between change in VO2 max and changes in E/A ratio .

Correlation between change in VO2 max and change in DT :

There was significant positive correlation between change in Vo2 max and change in DT as r = 0.349 and p < 0.05 as shown in figure 42.

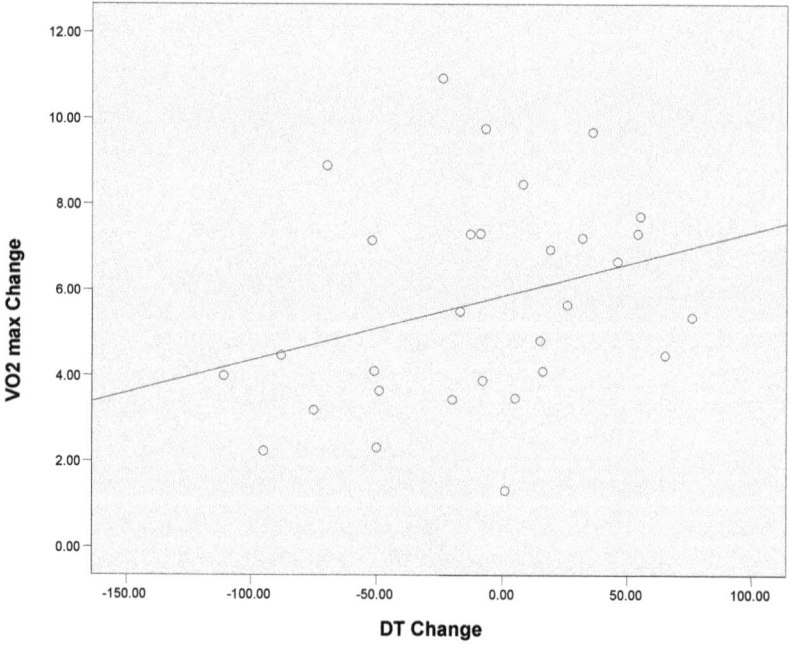

Figure 42: Correlations between change in VO2 max and change in DT

Discussion

Long term physical activities can cause some structural and functional changes in heart and this is called athlete's heart. General morphological changes consist of left ventricular (LV) dilatation, wall thickening, and increase in left ventricular mass. These alterations in sportsmen are physiological responses of increase in pressure or volume load. Symmetrical wall thickening and left ventricular widening without any changes in its shape can occur after regular physical exercise. This type of adaptation is called eccentric LV hypertrophy. Increase in ventricular wall thickness without any change in internal diameter is called concentric LV hypertrophy. Cardiac adaptations may differentiate according to the type of sport **(Ziya et al., 2011).**

In general, studies have proven that athletes participating in purely endurance sports such as long distance running and tennis are subject to chronic increases in cardiac preload which causes increase in stroke volume through increasing end diastolic volume, while those participating in purely resistance sports such as weightlifting and body-building tend to develop a large increase in LV wall thickness which increase stroke volume through decreasing end systolic volume **(Kuchynka et al., 2010).**

Volleyball has been classified as a moderate static and high dynamic sport, therefore involving a combination of resistance and endurance training **(Dzudie et al., 2007)**.

Direct measurement of maximum oxygen uptake (VO2max) is recognized as the best single index of aerobic fitness. However, the direct measurement of VO2max is difficult, exhausting, and often hazardous to perform regardless of the type of ergometer used. Because the direct testing procedure is rather complicated for larger populations, several indirect running and walking tests have been developed **(Chatterjee et al., 2011).**

Cardiac troponin T (cTnT) measured in serum or plasma is highly sensitive and specific markers of acute myocardial injury, and is recommended for the diagnosis of acute myocardial infarction **(Lowbeer et al., 2007).** In purely endurance sports such as marathon runners serum cTnT was reversibly elevated when measured just after finishing the race or within the first 24 hours **(Middleton et al., 2008).**

136

Our study aimed to study the ability of diastolic function measured by echocardiography to reflect changes in endurance as assessed by Vo2 max in response to combined strengthening and endurance training in male volleyball players and we tried to detect any subclinical cardiac changes by mean of serum cardiac troponin T in male volleyball players.

This study was conducted on 30 apparently healthy volleyball male players free from any medical or surgical illness, aging from 20-35 years and playing at Media Sporting Club and participating in the Egyptian volleyball league.

The players were all males, their mean age was 26.27 ± 4.25 years. Their mean weight was 85.20 ± 9.83 kg, while their mean height was 187.6 ± 7.27 cm and their mean BMI was 24.31 ± 1.79 Kg/m² as shown in table 1. Their mean systolic blood pressure (SBP) was 116.17 ± 7.27 mmHg while their diastolic blood pressure (DBP) was 77 ± 6.77 mmHg and their mean resting heart rate was 76.63 ± 8.04 beat/min as shown in table 2.

Our results were similar to **Naylor et al., 2005** who used echocardiography and Doppler imaging to assess left

137

ventricular (LV) dimensions and indices of diastolic filling in 22 elite athletes (rowing) at the end of their 'off-season' (baseline) and, subsequently, following 3 and 6 months of training. Their mean age were 20.4 ± 0.7 years, mean weight 81.5 ± 1.8 kg, mean height 186.2 ± 1.0 cm, mean (SBP) 122 ± 2 mmHg, mean (DBP) 78 ± 2 mmHg and their mean resting heart rate (HR) 56 ± 2 beat/min.

All these demographic data were similar to our values except for resting heart rate which was much lower than our study and this may be due to the difference in the sport activity where rowing which is also a combined sport (both endurance and resistive activity) has endurance more than volleyball.

As regards echocardiographic cardiac structure in our study, the mean left ventricular end diastolic dimension (LVEDD) was 53.7 ± 3.4 mm. Mean left ventricular end systolic dimension (LVESD) was 33.8 ± 3.7 mm , while the mean interventricular septal thickness (IVST) was 9.8 ± 0.9 mm .The mean posterior wall thickness (PWT) was 9.9 ± 0.8 while mean left ventricular mass index(LVMI) was 97.3 ± 15.5 gm/m^2 . All these values were within normal range for the same age and sex group as reported by **Barbier et al., 2006**, except LVESD which may be considered above normal in 3 players but **Thomson and Etes, 2007** reported that LVESD could reach up to 40 mm in endurance athletes. Also LVMI was higher than normal in 3 players and **Mayet et al., 2002** reported that LVMI may reach up to 141 gm/m^2 in endurance athletes with eccentric left ventricular hypertrophy and up to 155 gm/m^2 in athletes with concentric left ventricular hypertrophy.

Our results were similar to **Naylor et al., 2005** who found that athletes exhibited significantly higher LV mass . Three months of training further increased LV mass in athletes .These trends for increased mass persisted following 6 months of training. This study suggests that following a period of relative inactivity the rate of ventricular relaxation during early diastole may be slowed in athletes who exhibit ventricular hypertrophy, whilst resumption of training increases the speed of ventricular relaxation in the presence of further hypertrophy of the left ventricle.

Also our results came in accordance with **kneffel et al., 2007** who studied echocardiographic data and Vo2 max in athletic subjects where the number of the subjects were 346 divided into 3 groups (purely endurance athletes, ball games players and power athletes) they measured left ventricular (LV) diastolic wall thickness (WTd), internal diameter (LVIDd), muscle mass (MM), heart rate (HR), fractional shortening (FS) and E/A ratio, were investigated in the 346 young males (18–35 years, 291 athletes of various events and 55 nonathletic control subjects).

In a study by **Ziya et al., 2011** who aimed to evaluate left ventricular echocardiographic cardiac structure in athletes and sedentary controls. The study population consisted of 26 highly trained athletes (group I), the number of basketball players, volleyball players and handball players were 11, 7 and 8, respectively while group II were age, sex and body mass index (BMI) adjusted 23 control subjects. Using standard transthoracic echocardiographic measurements. There was a significant increase in LVEDD, LVESD, IVS and LVMI between group I and group II in the case of echocardiographic findings. They concluded that echocardiography techniques are novel and more sensitive and more effective methods and can be used to determine cardiac functions of athletes as a new tool and an efficient method.

On comparing our results of echocardiographic cardiac structure with the results of **Naylor et al., 2005** and **Ziya et al., 2011**, we found that they are nearly similar, taking in consideration that these measures were done at the period of off season after stoppage of training for 8 weeks in our study and 6 weeks in **Naylor et al., 2005** and during the training period in **Ziya et al., 2011** study.

On measuring echocardiographic systolic function in our study the mean stroke volume was 116.6 ± 20.9 ml, while mean ejection fraction (EF) was 65.7 ± 5.7 % and mean fractional shortening (FS) was 37 ± 4.9 .

All these values of systolic function are within normal range for the same age and sex group as reported by **Lang et al., 2005** except one player with FS equals 53.5 % before training which is above normal. In **Naylor et al., 2005** mean stroke volume (SV) was 95.05 ± 2.78 ml, mean EF was $70 \pm 1\%$ and mean FS 39 ± 1 %, all these values were before training and they did not compare between systolic function before and after training program.

In the current study echocardiographic diastolic function

showed mean propagation velocity (Vp) 64.1 ± 10.44 cm/sec. This value was within normal range for athletes in the same age and sex as reported by **Moller et al., 2000.** Mean Deceleration time (DT) was 180.8 ± 34.38 ms which was within normal range as stated by **Moller et al., 2000** except for 2 players where DT values were < 140 msec and this may be pseudonormal left ventricular filling pattern and is differentiated from restrictive diastolic dysfunction by Vp which is > 45 cm/sec according to **Moller et al., 2000.**

In our study echocardiographic mean E/A ratio was 1.64 ± 0.39 this value of E/A ratio was within normal range as found by **Gottdiener et al., 2004** except for 5 players where E/A were > 2 and this could be considered normal in athletes according to the explanation of **Green et al., 2006.**

We measured serum cardiac troponin T where the mean value was 0.06 ± 0.02 ng/ml and this value is above the minimal detection limit which is 0.01 ng/ml and below the level of 0.1 ng/ml, which is considered positive as stated by **Stolear et al., 1999.**

In our study maximal oxygen consumption Vo2 was

142

measured which is an indicator of endurance capacity of athletes. Its mean was 50.76 ± 6.91 ml/min/kg, this result was within expected values for this group as reported by **Wilmore and Costill, 2005.**

Kneffel et al., 2007 studied Vo2 max in athletic subjects where the number of the subjects were 346 divided into 3 groups (purely endurance athletes, ball games players and power athletes VO2max was measured. Their mean Vo2 max was 70 ± 6.7 ml/min/kg for endurance athletes, 62.9 ± 6.8 for combined athletes and 55 ± 8.9 for power athletes.

When the groups were pooled results indicate that in athletes having higher endurance capacity maximal oxygen consumption depends largely on cardiac condition, while in athletes with a lower endurance capacity it can be limited by peripheral conditions. It is important to notice that in the previous study it is not clear when these data were taken during the training cycle, also there is difference in competition level between players in our study and players in **Kneffel et al., 2007.**

A training program was designed in the form of combined strengthening and endurance exercises with frequency of

143

training 6 times/week for 12 weeks in the form of three days strengthening exercise alternating with another three days of endurance exercises, each training session was 45-60 minutes. Then we measured the echocardiographic cardiac structure, systolic function and the diastolic function, we also we measured serum cardiac troponin T and the maximum oxygen consumption (Vo2 max) .

In our study we Compared between echocardiographic cardiac structure before and after training and there was significant increase in IVST and PWT where t = -3.889 and -3.798 respectively and p < 0.005 and significant decrease in LVEDD where t = 2.546 and p< 0.05 while there were no significant differences in LVESD and LVMI before and after training.

In the study of **Naylor et al., (2005)** who found significant increased measures of cardiac structure in athletes in the form of increased IVST, PWT, LVMI, and LVESD and there were no change in LVEDD following 3 months of training, these findings were also evident following 6 months. These results were nearly similar to our results taking in consideration that

144

subjects in this study practiced a combined training program as in our study.

Our results were nearly similar to results of **Rodrigues et al., 2006** who aimed to study the cardiovascular changes occurring in response to endurance training in young men by assessing the effects of 6 months of moderate-intensity aerobic training (1 hour/day, 3 times/week) on normal hearts, 23 men were studied by standard and tissue Doppler echocardiography. They found increase in IVST, PWT and LVMI while there were no significant increase in LVEDD and LVESD.

In a study by **Baggish et al., 2007** who studied the effect of participation in team-based exercise training on cardiac structure and function. Competitive endurance athletes and strength athletes were studied with echocardiography at baseline and after 90 days of team training. They found that endurance athletes experienced significant increase in LVESD, LVEDD and LVMI with biatrial enlargement and biventricular dilation with an accompanying enhancement in biventricular function. In contrast, strength athletes demonstrated increased IVST, PWT and LVMI with concentric LV hypertrophy with diminished LV diastolic function. The longitudinal data from

145

this study provide convincing evidence that athletic training has a causal role in the development of training-specific profiles of cardiac structure and function. The difference between this study and our study is that the subjects were divided into endurance athletes and strength athletes while in our study they were one group of combined athletes (volleyball).

In our study we compared between echocardiographic systolic function before and after training and we found significant difference in SV where $t = 3.668$ and $p < 0.005$. And there were significant differences in FS and EF before and after training where $t = 2.714$ and 2.350 respectively and $p<0.05$ this indicate that all indices of systolic function decreases after training program .

Our results were nearly similar to **Rodrigues et al., 2006** who aimed to study the cardiovascular changes occurring in response to endurance training in young men and they found no change in ejection fraction and stroke volume after training.

Also in the study of **Baggish et al., 2007** who studied the effect of participation in team-based exercise training on cardiac structure and function. Competitive endurance athletes and strength athletes were studied with echocardiography at baseline and after 90 days of team training. They found no significance change in EF and FS in both endurance and strength athletes.

Same results were also found by **Mantziari et al., 2010** who examined left ventricular (LV) function in elite young athletes in relation to structural adaptation to prolonged intense training. Conventional echocardiography and tissue Doppler imaging (TDI) were performed in 15 elite rowers and 12 sedentary matched controls, they found significant decrease in FS between the athletes and the sedentary subjects while there were no significant difference in the EF between the 2 groups.

Moreover similar results were found by **Abergel et al., 2011** who examined 22 male runners in 2008 and 23 male runners in 2009 they have an echocardiography the day before the race and after the race. They measured ejection fraction (EF) LV fractional shortening (FS) and end systolic stress (ESS). They found significant decrease in EF and FS indicating decrease in the systolic function after long distance running.

Our results were nearly similar to **Rodrigues et al., 2006, baggish et al., 2007** and **Abergel et al., 2011** which were all prospective studies as our study also similar to the cross-sectional study by **Mantziari et al., 2010.**

As regard the comparison between echocardiographic diastolic function before and after training and we found highly significant difference as regard propagation velocity Vp before and after training program where t = -9.186 and p< 0.005. On the other hand there were no significant differences in E/A ratio and DT before and after training where t = 1.144 and 1.054 respectively and p > 0.05 .

Exactly same results were found **Naylor et al., 2005** who found increase in Vp at base line and following 3 months of training while there were no difference in deceleration time DT and in E/A ratio.

Our results as regards propagation velocity was the only parameter of diastolic function which significantly improved after training these findings come in accordance with study by **Tumuklu et al., 2007** who compared tissue Doppler imaging TDI and Vp findings in professional football players and age-adjusted sedentary controls to assess the effect of regular athletic training on myocardial function. They found significant improvement in left ventricular diastolic function that can be detected by significant improvement of Vp while there were no significant improvement of E/A ratio and they did not measure deceleration time DT.

Also similar results were reported in a study by **Popovic et al., 2011** who used standard and tissue Doppler to assess cardiac parameters in 16 elite male wrestlers (strength training), 21 water polo player (endurance training), and 20 sedentary subjects of similar age. They found no significant difference in E/A ratio and DT between the 2 groups or between each group and the control group.

In the current study we were pioneer in measuring serum cardiac troponin T at the off season period before training and another time after the training program and there was no significant difference between the two readings where t = -0.733 and p> 0.05 .

In the study by **Middleton et al., 2008** who measured cTnT release during and after completion of a marathon using repeated blood draws. Nine well-trained men completed a marathon (42.2 km) on a motorized treadmill. Measures were done at rest and at 30-min intervals during, immediately after, and at 1, 3, 6,12, and 24 h after exercise. They found reversible increase in serum cTnT during the race and after one hour and all levels returned to baseline after one hour. They concluded that minor elevations in cTnT subsequent to endurance exercise are due reversible cardiomyocyte membrane damage that may reflect part of a remodeling process. Although cTnT is diagnostic of acute coronary syndrome in the clinical setting, in a healthy exercising population, cTnT is routinely released in all persons after periods of increased myocardial demand.

Recently **Carranza-García et al., 2011** examined the acute effect of a heavy resistance training session (n=18 males) and an indoor soccer match (n=21, 11 males, 10 females) on the release of cTnI, cTnT, and NT-proBNP. Blood samples collected at rest, immediately post- and at 1, 3, 6, 12, and 24 h post-exercise. They found That heavy resistance training session resulted in an increase in NT-proBNP but not in cTnI or cTnT. The indoor soccer match led to an increase in the release of NT-proBNP and cTnT in both males and females but not cTnI. They concluded that intermittent bouts of exercise result in only modest release of cardiac biomarkers with very limited evidence of myocyte injury.

To our knowledge our study was the only study that measured serum cTnT at rest and after a designed training program, all the previous studies as **Middleton et al., 2008** and **Carranza-García et al., 2011** assessed serum cTnT during or just after the exercise bout, also **Mousavi et al., 2009** and **Mingels et al., 2009** reported reversible elevation of serum cTnT and attributed it to cytosolic release of the biomarker, not to the true breakdown of the cardiomyocyte.

We measured maximal oxygen consumption Vo2 max before and after the training program and there was highly significant difference in the two readings with t= -12.72 and p< 0.001 .

Our results were similar to **Naylor et al., 2005,** they found significant increase in vo2 max at base line and following 3 months of training and there was further increase following 6 months of training.

151

Recently **Rankovic et al., 2010** measured absolute and relative VO2 max in 66 male subjects. Subjects were divided into two groups of active athletes (football players (n=22) and volleyball players (n=19), while the third group of non-athletes served as control group (n=26). They aimed to analyze the aerobic capacity as an indicator of physical capacity of athletes and to determine differences in their aerobic capacity with regard to the kind of sport they are practicing, as well as the differences obtained when compared to physically inactive subjects. Their results showed that football players have higher Vo2 max followed by volleyball players followed by non athletes. They concluded that football as a sport requires higher degree of endurance compared to volleyball also Vo2 max is higher in the groups of athletes compared to the group of non-athletes. These results we nearly similar to ours but Vo2 max in our results was higher than volleyball players in this study because of the difference in competition level.

Moreover similar data were reported by **Helgerud et al., 2010** who studied the effect of 8 weeks of combined strength and endurance training on 21 first league elite football players having recently participated in the UEFA Champions League. They found that VO2 max increased 8.6 %, from 60.5 to 65.7 ml/min/kg.

In our study, we started to correlate between demographic data and diastolic function before training where we found significant positive correlation between age and propagation velocity (Vp) before training as r = 0.486 and p< 0.05. While there were no significant correlation between age and E/A and between age and DT .

Also we found significant positive correlation between body mass index (BMI) and deceleration time (DT) (indicating decrease in the diastolic function) before training with r = 0.363 and p < 0.05. While there were no significant correlation between BMI and E/A ratio and between BMI and propagation velocity (Vp) before training .

Similarly **Russo et al., 2011** assessed the effect of increased body size on left ventricular diastolic function by evaluating left ventricular diastolic function in 950 participants by traditional and tissue Doppler imaging. Peak early transmitral diastolic flow velocity (E) and late transmitral diastolic flow velocity (A) was evaluated and E/A was calculated. The study sample was divided into 3 groups: normal weight (BMI< 25.0 kg/m2), overweight (BMI = 25.0 to 29.9 kg/m2), and obese (BMI >30 kg/m2). They found significant negative correlation between BMI and E/A ratio and this indicates that increase in BMI may be associated with decrease in diastolic function of impaired relaxation pattern which is manifested by decrease in E/A ratio and increase in DT .

When comparing our results with those of **Russo et al., 2011** they were similar in that increase in BMI is associated with decrease in diastolic function which is manifested by increase in DT in our study and by decrease in E/A ratio in **Russo et al., 2011** study.

We correlated between demographic data and Vo2 max before training where we found significant negative correlation between BMI and Vo2 max before training with r = -0.406 and p < 0.05. The same result was also reported by **Cho et al., 2010** who investigated the combined effect of body mass index (BMI) and physical fitness on serum vaspin in Korean young men. They examined 490 Korean men and found highly significant negative correlation between BMI and Vo2 max.

In the current study correlation between Vo2 max and diastolic function before training was significantly positive as $r = 0.413$ and $p < 0.05$. While there were no significant correlation between Vo2 max and E/A ratio and DT before training.

Also and there was significant positive correlation between Vo2 max and E/A ratio after training ($r = 0.325$ and $p < 0.05$), and there was significant positive correlation between Vo2 max and Vp after training ($r = 0.318$ and $p < 0.05$). From our results we can figure that Vp is the only parameter of diastolic function that correlate with Vo2 max before and after training.

In a study by **Vinereanu et al., 2002** they studied 18 endurance-trained and 11 strength-trained athletes and compared them with 14 sedentary controls. Global systolic function and diastolic function were measured, also maximal oxygen consumption was measured. They found positive correlation between Vo2 max and E/A ratio in the endurance group but not in strength trained athletes also there was no significant correlation between Vo2 max and Vp. They concluded that endurance-trained athletes had higher left ventricular diastolic function and that dynamic exercise training improves cardiac performance by an effect on diastolic function.

Also **kneffel et al., 2007** studied Vo2 max in athletic subjects who were divided into 3 groups (purely endurance athletes, ball games players and power athletes) they found highly significant positive correlation between Vo2 max and E/A ratio in all three groups but they did not measure DT and Vp. These results were similar to our results in that both studies confirms that increase in physical fitness is associated with increase in diastolic function taking in consideration that **kneffel et al.,** perform their study during the middle of the training cycle.

Our results come in accordance with the results of **Vinereanu et al., 2002** in that there is close relation between physical fitness and diastolic function but in our study the main parameter to determine this was Vp while in **Vinereanu et al., 2002** and **kneffel et al., 2007** the E/A was the main parameter to determine this. Both studies relied on the E/A ratio, which has several limitations including the preload dependence while Vp is better indicator of diastolic function because it is relatively insensitive to changes in preload

156

compared to E/A ratio **(Gottdiener et al., 2004).**

Correlation between changes in Vo2 max and changes in diastolic function (Vp, E/A and DT) showed significant positive correlation between change in Vo2 max and changes in Vp (r= 0.351 and p < 0.05) and significant positive correlation between change in Vo2 max and changes in E/A ratio (r= 0.372 and p < 0.05) and significant positive correlation between change in Vo2 max and changes in Vp (r = 0.349 and p < 0.05).

Nearly similar results was reported by **Stewart et al., 2006** who studied the effect of combined training program for 6 months on 51 subjects, they assessed Cardiac size , LV diastolic function, maximum oxygen consumption (VO2 max), muscle strength and general and abdominal fatness. They found positive correlation between changes in Vo2 max and changes in E/A ratio but not changes in Vp. These findings were similar to our finding when correlating between changes inVo2 max with changes in E/A ratio, but not in changes in Vp and this may be due to difference in age group studied.

While in another study by **Andersen et al., 2010**, who examined the cardiac effects of football training (n= 19) and

157

running (n= 18) for 16 weeks in inactive women by echocardiography . They found significant increase in the Vo2 max as well as in the diastolic function after training in both group but correlations between change in Vo2 max and changes in diastolic function were not studied.

In summary we found that combined training program lead to significant increase in cardiac wall thickness, diastolic function of the heart (mainly Vp) and in maximal oxygen consumption (Vo2 max), also we found that there is a close relation between changes in Vo2 max and changes in all indices of diastolic function studied (Vp, E/A ratio and DT).

Summary and conclusion

Long-term athletic training is associated with cardiac changes including increased left ventricular (LV) cavity dimension, wall thickness, and calculated mass that have been extensively studied and are commonly described as ''athlete's heart'' (**Spirito et al., 1994).**

In general, studies have proven that athletes participating in purely endurance sports such as long distance running and tennis are subjected to chronic increases in cardiac preload which causes increase in stroke volume through increasing end diastolic volume, while those participating in purely resistance sports such as weightlifting and body-building tend to develop a large increase in LV wall thickness which increase stroke volume through decreasing end systolic volume **(Fagard 2003)**.

A commonly used method to investigate endurance capacity is the measurement of the maximal oxygen uptake by spiroergometry. It can therefore be assumed that spiroergometrically measured maximal oxygen consumption will correlate with various attributes of the athlete's heart as an

159

important   determinant   of   aerobic   performance **(Kneffel et al., 2007).**

VO2 max has been defined as: "the highest rate of oxygen consumption attainable during maximal or exhaustive exercise" As exercise intensity increases, so does oxygen consumption. However, a point is reached where exercise intensity can continue to increase without the associated rise in oxygen consumption **(Wilmore and Costill 2005).**

Our study aimed to study the ability of diastolic function measured by echocardiography to reflect changes in endurance as assessed by Vo2 max in response to combined strengthening and endurance training in male volleyball players and we tried to detect any subclinical cardiac changes by mean of serum cardiac troponin T in male volleyball players.

This study was conducted on 30 apparently healthy volleyball male players free from any medical or surgical illness, aging from 20-35 years and playing at Media Sporting Club and participating in the Egyptian volleyball league.

160

The study started at the beginning of the training cycle after stoppage of training for at least 8 weeks, after routine history taking and general examination echocardiography was done to all players where we measured cardiac structure,

systolic function and diastolic function. Vo2 max was also calculated by ergospirometry and serum cardiac troponin T was measured.

A combined training program was designed for 12 weeks after that echocardiography, vo2 max and serum cardiac troponin T was repeated.

we found that combined training program lead to significant increase in cardiac wall thickness, diastolic function of the heart (mainly Vp) and in maximal oxygen consumption (Vo2 max), also we found that there is a close relation between changes in Vo2 max and changes in all indices of diastolic function studied (Vp, E/A ratio and DT).

We concluded that Diastolic function measured by echocardiography mainly propagation velocity (Vp), E/A ratio and deceleration time (DT) can reflect changes in endurance as

161

previously assessed by Vo2 max only, in response to combined strengthening and endurance training program. Moreover, Vp is better indicator of diastolic function in athletes than E/A ratio and DT.

Echocardiographic parameters of cardiac hypertrophy mainly interventricular septal thickness (IVS), posterior wall thickness (PWT) and left ventricular end diastolic dimension (LVEDD) increase in response to combined training program. This increase is accompanied by improved LV diastolic function suggesting a physiological rather than a pathological cardiac hypertrophy.

As a result, we suggest that echocardiographic techniques are novel , more sensitive and more effective methods to determine cardiac functions and dimension in athletes performing combined endurance and strengthening training as a new efficient tool.

On the other hand, we did not find any role for serum cardiac troponin T in detecting subclinical cardiac changes in athletes when measured before and after combined endurance and strengthening training program.

Recommendation

1. Using echocardiographic diastolic function mainly Vp as a specific diagnostic tool to assess endurance in athletes in the preseason screening and to evaluate the efficiency of any training program containing endurance exercise.

2. More studies on the type of cardiac hypertrophy in response to different training stimuli.

3. Measuring Vo2 max as an indicator of endurance in athletes especially before recruitment in a training cycle.

4. Performing more studies on serum cardiac enzymes other than cardiac troponin as CK-MB, LDH, SGOT and myoglobin to detect any subclinical cardiac injury and differentiate between physiological and pathological cardiac hypertrophy in athletes.

.

References

Abergel E, Chatellier G and Hagege A. (2004): Serial left ventricular adaptations in world-class professional cyclists: implications for disease screening and follow-up. J Am Coll Cardiol; 44:144–9.

Abergel E, Simon M, Bogino E, Jimene M and Chauve C (2011): Left ventricular systolic function is not accurately evaluated by left ventricular ejection after a long distance running. Archives of Cardiovascular Diseases, Volume 10ion fract4, Issue 4, April 2011, Pages 298-299.

Andersen L, Hansen P, Sogaard P Madsen J. Bech J and Krustrup P.(2010): Improvement of systolic and diastolic heart function after physical training in sedentary women. Scand J Med Sci Sports 2010: 20 (Suppl. 1): 50–573.

Baggish A, Wang F, Weiner R, Elinoff J, Tournoux F, Boland A, Picard M, Hutter A and Malissa J.(2008): Training-specific changes in cardiac structure and function: a prospective and longitudinal assessment of competitive athletes . J Appl Physiol 104:1121-1128.

Barbier J, Lebiller E and Ville N. (2006): Relationships between sports specific characteristics of athlete's heart and maximal oxygen uptake. Eur J Cardiovasc Prev Rehabil; 13: 115–21.

Barbier J, Ville N, Kervio G, Walther G and Carré F. (2006): Sports-Specific Features of Athlete's Heart and their Relation to Echocardiographic Parameters. Herz 31 · Nr. 6 Urban & Vogel,531-543.

Barry J, Maron MD and Pelliccia A. (2006): The Heart of Trained Athletes Cardiac Remodeling and the Risks of Sports, Including Sudden Death. Circulation; 114; 1633-1644.

Basavarajaiah S, Wilson M, Whyte G, Shah A, McKenna W,and Sharma S. (2008): Prevalence of hypertrophic cardiomyopathy in highly trained athletes. J Am Coll Cardiol; 51:1033–9.

Basso C, Thiene G, Corrado D, Buja G, Melacini P and Nava (2000): Hypertrophic cardiomyopathy and sudden death in the young: pathologic evidence of myocardial ischemia. Hum Pathol. 2000 Aug;31(8):988-98

Braunwald E, Antman EM, Beasley JW, Califf RM, Cheitlin MD, Hochman. (2002): Guideline update for the management of patients with unstable angina and non-ST-segment elevation myocardial infarction. J Am Coll Cardiol.;40:1366-74.

Bryant C and Peterson J (2001): Muscular strength and endurance: ACSM's Resource Manual for Guidelines for Exercise Testing and Prescription. Philadelphia, PA, Lipppincott Williams & Wilkins.

Bssavarajaiah S, Boraita A, and Whyte G (2008): Ethnic differences in left ventricular remodeling in highly-trained athletes. Relevance to differentiating physiologic left ventricular hypertrophy from hypertrophic cardiomyopathy. J Am Coll Cardiol; 51:2256–62.

Burke AP, Farb V, Virmani R, Goodin J and Smialek JE. (1991): Sports-related and non-sports-related sudden cardiac death in young adults. Am Heart J.; 121:568 –575.

Campos GE, Luecke TJ and Wendeln HK (2002): Muscular adaptations in response to three different resistance training regimens: Specificity of repetition maximum training zones. Eur

J Appl Physiol 88:50–60.

Carranza-García LE, George K, Serrano-Ostáriz E, Casado-Arroyo R, Caballero-Navarro AL and Legaz-Arrese A (2011): Cardiac biomarker response to intermittent exercise bouts. Int J Sports Med. 2011 May;32(5):327-31.

Chatterjee P, Banerjee A and Das P (2011): A Prediction Equation to Estimate the Maximum Oxygen Uptake of School-Age Girls from Kolkata, India. Malays J Med Sci. Jan-Mar;18(1):25-29.

Chee CE, Anastassiades CP, Antonopoulos AG, Petsas AA and Anastassiades LC (2005): Cardiac hypertrophy and how it may break an athlete's heart the Cypriot case. Eur J Echocardiogr;6:301-7.

Cheng TO (1990): Hypertrophic cardiomyopathy evolving into a hypokinetic and dilated left ventricle: coronary embolization as a probable pathogenetic mechanism. Clin Cardiol;13(10):A31.

Cheng TO (2001): Valsalva maneuver is not a held deep

inspiration. Am J Cardiol; 88:1219–20.

Cheng TO (2007): The evolution of cardiology in China. Cardiothoracic surgery in China: past, present and future. Hong Kong: The Chinese University of Hong Kong;. p. 204–305.

Cheng TO (2008): Hypertrophic cardiomyopathy in China: from bench to bedside. Int J Cardiol Nov. 12; 130:121–4.

Cheng TO (2009): Hypertrophic cardiomyopathy vs athlete's heart. International Journal of Cardiology 131 (2009) 151–155.

Cho JK, Han TK and Kang HS (2010): Combined effects of body mass index and cardio/respiratory fitness on serum vaspin concentrations in Korean young men. Eur J Appl Physiol , 108:347–353.

Claessens P, Claessens C and Claessens M (2004): Cardiac function by strain imaging: Key to the increased performance capacities of endurance-trained athletes. Echocardiography;21:204–205.

Corrado D, Basso C, Pavei A, Schiavon M and Thiene G (2005): Decline of sudden cardiac death in young competitive athletes after implementation of Italian preparticipation screening. Circulation.; 112(suppl II):II-831–II-832. Abstract.

Corrado D, Basso C, Rizzoli G and Thiene G. (2003): Does sport activity enhance the risk of sudden death in adolescents and young adults? J Am Coll Cardiol.; 42:1964 –1966.

Corrado D, Basso C, Schiavon M and Thiene G (1998): Screening for hypertrophic cardiomyopathy in young athletes. N Engl J Med.; 339:364 –369.

D'Andrea A, Caso P and Severino S (2006): Prognostic value of intra-left ventricular electromechanical asynchrony in patients with hypertrophic cardiomyopathy. Eu Heart J 2006; 27:1311–8.

Darren R, Warburton A, William S And Mckenzie D (2008): Chapter 2, Cardiorespiratory adaptations to training, Olympic textbook of medicine in sport.

Demaree S, Powers S and Lawler J (2001): Fundamentals of exercise metabolism ACSM's 82 SECTION 1 • General Considerations In Sports Medicine Chapter 14 • Nutrition 83.Resource Manual for Exercise Testing and Prescription. Philadelphia, PA, Lipincott Williams & Wilkins.

Deuster PA and Keyser DO (2005): Sport medicine just the facts, Section 1 general considerations in sport medicine, chapter 8 Basics In Exercise Physiology.

Dickhuth HH, Roecker K and Niess A (1996): The echocardiographic determination of volume and muscle mass of the heart. Int J Sports Med; 17: Suppl 3:S132–9.

Donal E, Rozoy T, Kervio G, Schnell F, Mabo F and Carré F (2011) : Comparison of the Heart Function Adaptation in Trained and Sedentary Men After 50 and Before 35 Years of Age. The American Journal of Cardiology, In Press, Corrected Proof, Available online 23 July 2011.

Duman D, Tokay S and Toprak A (2005): Elevated cardiac troponin T is associated with increased left ventricular mass index and predicts mortality in continuous ambulatory peritoneal dialysis patients. Nephrol Dial Transplant;20(5):962—7.

171

Durstine J, Davis P, Roitman J, Haver E and Herridge M (2001): Specificity of exercise training and testing, ACSM's Resource , Manual for Guidelines for Exercise Testing and Prescription. Philadelphia, PA, Lipppincott Williams & Wilkins. echocardiography. J Am Coll Cardiol 1986; 7: 190-203.

Dzudie A, Menanga A, Hamadou B, Atchou G and Kingue S (2007): Ultrasonographic study of left ventricular function at rest in a group of highly trained black African handball players. Eur J Echocardiography 8, 122-127.

Erol MK and Karakelleoglu S (2002): Assessment of right heart function in the athlete's heart. Heart Vessels; 16:175–80.

Fagard R (2003): Athlete's heart. Heart;89:1455-61.

Fleck SJ and Kraemer WJ (2004): Designing resistance training programs, 3rd edn. Human Kinetics, Champaign, IL, USA.

Franklin B, Roitman J, Haver E and Herridge M (2001): Normal cadiorespiratory responses to acute aerobic exercise : ACSM's Resource Manual for Guidelines for Exercise Testing and Prescription. Philadelphia, PA, Lippincott Williams & Wilkins.

Franklin B, Whaley M and Howley E (2000): Benefits and risks associated with exercise: ACSM's Guidlines for Exercise Testing and Prescription. Philadelphia, PA, Lippincott Williams & Willliams.

Franklin B, Whaley M and Howley E (2000): General principles of exercise prescription: ACSM's Guidelines for Exercise Testing and Prescription. Philadelphia, PA, Lippincott Williams & Wilkins.

Franklin B, Whaley M and Howley E (2000): Health screening and risking stratification: ACSM's Guidelines for Exercise Testing and Prescription. Philadelphia, PA, Lippincott Williams & Williams.

Franklin B, Whaley M and Howley E (2000): Physical fitness testing and interpretation: ACSM's Guidelines for Exercise Testing and Prescription. Philadelphia, PA, Lippincott Williams & Wilkins.

Fredette D, Roitman J and Haver E (2001): Exercise Recommendations for Flexibility and Range of Motion: ACSM's Resource Manual for Guidelines for Exercise Testing and Prescription, Philadelphia, PA, Lipppincott Williams & Wilkins.

George KP, Gates PE, Whyte G and Lea R (1999): Echocardiographic examination of cardiac structure and function in elite cross trained male and female alpine skiers. Br J Sports Med. 1999;33:93–99.

Godon P, Griffet V, Vinsonneau U, Caignault JR, Prevosto JM, Quiniou G, Guerard S (2009): Athlete's heart or hypertrophic cardiomyopathy: usefulness of N-terminal pro-brain natriuretic peptide. Int J Cardiol. Sep 11;137(1):72-4. Epub 2008 Aug 3.

Goodman M, Liu P & Green J (2005): Left ventricular adaptations following short-term endurance training. Journal of Applied Physiology 98, 454–460.

Gottdiener J, Bednarz J, Gardin J, Klein A, Manning W and Weissman N (2004): American society of echocardiography recommendations for use of echocardiography in clinical trials. J am soc echo 17, 1086-119.

Green D, Naylor L and George K (2006): Cardiac and vascular adaptations to exercise. Curr Opin Clin Nutr Metab Care 9:677–684.

Griffet V, Guérard S, Galoisy-Guibal L, Caignault JR, Bernard F and Brion R (2007): Normal values of the peak early diastolic Ea using myocardial tissue Doppler in 100 elite athletes. Arch Mal Coeur Vaiss; 100:809–15.

Helgerud J, Rodas G, Kemi OJ and Hoff J (2010): Strength and endurance in elite football players. Int J Sports Med. Sep;32(9):677-82.

Henriksen E, Landelius J and Wesslen L. (1996): Echocardiographic right and left ventricular measurements in male elite endurance athletes. Eur Heart J; 17:1121–8.

Hoit B (2007): Left ventricular diastolic function. Crit Care Med Vol. 35, No. 8 (Suppl.).

Holly R and Shaffrath J (2001): Cardiorespiratory Endurance: ACSM's Resource Manual for Guidelines for Exercise Testing and Prescription. Philadelphia,PA, Lippincott Williams & Wilkins.

Humphrey R (2001): Musculoskeletal anatomy : ACSM's Resource Manual for Guidelines for Exercise Testing and Prescription. Philadelphia, PA, Lipincott Williams & Wilkins.

Iglesias-Cubero G, Batalla A and Rodriguez Reguero J (2000): Left ventricular mass index and sports: the influence of different sports activities and arterial blood pressure. Int J Cardiol; 75:261–5.

Jeremias A and Gibson CM (2005): Narrative review: alternative causes for elevated cardiac troponin levels when acute coronary syndromes are excluded. Ann Intern Med;142(9):786—91.

Karvonin M, Kentala k and Mustala O (1957): The effects of training heart rate; A longitudinal study. Ann med exp boil fenn ; 35 : 307- 15.

Kasapis C and Thompson P (2008): Olympic Textbook Of Medicine In Sport Sports Cardiology.

Kingue S, Binam F and Atchou G (2001): chocardiographique. de la fonction ventriculaire gauche d'un groupe de judokas camerounais. Sciences Sports;16:10-5.

Klues HG, Schiffers A, and Maron BJ (1995): Phenotypic spectrum and patterns of left ventricular hypertrophy in hypertrophic cardiomyopathy: morphologic observations and significance as assessed by twodimensional echocardiography in 600 patients. J Am Coll Cardiol; 26:1699–708.

Kneffel Z, Horvath P, Petrekanits M, N´emeth H, Sido Z, and Pavlik G (2007): Relationship between Relative Aerobic Power and Echocardiographic Characteristics in Male Athletes. Echocardiography Vol. 24, No. 9.

Knuttgen G (2003): The science of exercise physiology: What is exercise? Phys. Sportsmed. 31(March):31–49.

Knuttgen G (2007): Strength Training And Aerobic Exercise: Comparison And Contrast. Journal of Strength and Conditioning

Research, 2007, 21(3), 973–978.

Kraemer J (2003): Strength training basics: Designing workouts to meet patient's goals. Phys. Sportsmed. 31(August):39–45.

Kraemer J and Hakkinen K (2002): Strength Training for Sport. Oxford:Blackwell Publishing.

Krieg A, Scharhag J, Kindermann W,and Urhausen A (2007): Cardiac tissue Doppler imaging in sports medicine. Sports Med; 37:15–30.

Kuchynka P, Palecek T, Vilikus Z, Havranek S, and Taborska K (2010): Cardiac Structural and Functional Changes in Competitive Amateur Cyclists. Echocardiography 2010;27:11-16

Lang RM, Bierig M, Devereux RB, Flachskampf FA, Foster E, Pellikka PA, Picard MH, Roman MJ, Seward J, Shanewise JS, Solomon SD, Spencer KT, Sutton MS and Stewart WJ.(2005) : Chamber Quantification Writing Group; American Society of Echocardiography's Guidelines and

178

standards Committee; European Association of Echocardiography. J Am Soc Echocardiogr. 2005 Dec;18(12):1440-63.

Libonati JR (1999): Myocardial diastolic function and exercise. Med Sci Sports Ex ; 31:1741–1747.

Link MS, Wang PJ, Pandian NG, Bharati S, Udelson JE, Lee M-Y ,Vecchiotti MA, VanderBrink BA, Mirra G, Maron BJ and Estes N (1998): An experimental model of sudden death due to low-energy chest-wall impact (commotio cordis). N Engl J Med.; 338:1805–1811.

Louise H, Leonard F, Jenny A, Playford D, maurogiovanni A, and Driscoll G (2005): Reduced ventricular flow propagation velocity in elite athletes is augmented with resumption of exercise training. J physiology pp 957-963.

Lowbeer C, Gustafsson SA and Seeberger A (2004): Serum cardiac troponin T in patients hospitalized with heart failure is associated with left ventricular hypertrophy and systolic dysfunction. Scand J Clin Lab Invest;64(7): 667—76.

Lowbeer C, Seebergerb A, Gustafsson S, Bouvier F and

Hulting J (2007): Serum cardiac troponin T, troponin I, plasma BNP and left ventricular mass index in professional football players. J Sci Med Sport. Oct;10(5):291-6. Epub 2007 Feb 6.

Hulting J (2007): Serum cardiac troponin T, troponin I, plasma BNP and left ventricular mass index in professional football players. Journal of Science and Medicine in Sport, 10, 291—296.

Ma JZ, Dai J, Sun B, Ji P, Yang D,and Zhang JN (2007): Cardiovascular preparticipation screening of young competitive athletes for prevention of sudden death in China. J Sci Med Sport; 10:227–33.

Magalski A, Maron BJ,and Main ML (2008): Relation of race to lectrocardiographic patterns in elite American football players. J Am Coll Cardiol; 51:2250–5.

Mantziari A,Vassilikos P, Giannakoulas G, Karamitsos T, Dakos G and Papadopoulou N (2010): Left ventricular function in elite rowers in relation to traininginduced structural myocardial adaptation. Scand J Med Sci Sports 2010: 20: 428–433.

Maron BJ and Zipes DP (2005): 36th Bethesda Conference. Introduction: Eligibility recommendations for competitive athletes with cardiovascular abnormalitiesgeneral considerations. J Am Coll Cardiol; 45:1318–21.

Maron BJ and Zipes DP (2005): 36th Bethesda Conference: eligibility recommendations for competitive athletes with cardiovascular abnormalities. J Am Coll Cardiol.; 45:1312–1375.

Maron BJ, Gohman TE, Kyle SB, Estes NAM and Link MS (2002): Clinical profile and spectrum of commotio cordis. JAMA.; 287:1142–1146.

Maron BJ, Gottdiener JS,and Epstein SE (1981): Patterns and significance of distribution of left ventricular hypertrophy in hypertrophic cardiomyopathy: a wide angle, two-dimensional echocardiographic study of 125 patients. Am J Card; 48:418–28.

Maron BJ, Pelliccia A, Spataro A,and Granata M (1993): Reduction in left ventricular wall thickness after deconditioning in highly trained Olympic athletes. Br Heart J; 69:125–8.

Maron BJ, Seidman JG,and Seidman CE (2004): Proposal for contemporary screening strategies in families with hypertrophic cardiomyopathy. J Am Coll Cardiol; 44:2125–32.

Maron BJ, Thompson PD, Puffer JC, McGrew CA, Strong WB, Douglas PS, Clark LT, Mitten MJ, Crawford MH, Atkins DL, Driscoll DJ and Epstein AE (1996): American Heart Association statement for health professionals: cardiovascular preparticipation screening of competitive athletes. Circulation.; 94:850–856.

Maron BJ (2002): Hypertrophic cardiomyopathy: a systematic review. JAMA; 287:1308–20.

Maron BJ (2003): Sudden death in young athletes. N Engl J Med.; 349: 1064–1075.

Maron BJ (2005): How should we screen competitive athletes for cardiovascular disease? Eur Heart J.; 26:428–430.

Mayet J, Ariff B, Wasan B, And Chapman N (2007): Midwall myocardial shortening in athletic left ventricular hypertrophy. International journal of cardiology. Vol 86, issue 2, page 233-238.

Middleton N, George K, Whyte D. Collinson G and Shave R (2008) : Cardiac troponin T release is stimulated by endurance exercise in healthy humans, J Am Coll Cardiol 52 , pp. 1813–1814.

Mingels A, Jacobs L, Michielsen E, Swaanenburg J, Wodzig W and van Dieijen-Visser M (2009): Reference population and marathon runner sera assessed by highly sensitive cardiac troponin T and commercial cardiac troponin T and I assays, Clin Chem 55.

Mitchell JH, Haskell W and Snell P (2005): Task Force 8: Classification of Sports. J Am Coll Cardiol; 8:1364–7.

Moller JE, Sondergaard E, Poulsen SH and Egstrup, K (2000): Left ventricular diastolic dysfunction is a predictor of outcome after a myocardial infarction. J Am Coll Cardiol; 36:1841.

Moller JE, Sondergaard E, Poulsen SH and Egstrup KJ

(2000): Reprinted with permission from the American College of Cardiology. Am Coll Cardiol ; 36:1841.

Morganroth J and Maron BJ (1977): The athlete's heart syndrome: a new perspective. Ann NY Acad Sci 1977; 301 (1): 931-41.

Morganroth J, Maron BJ and Henry WL (1975): Comparative left ventricular dimensions in trained athletes. Ann Intern Med; 81:1001–4.

Mousavi N, Czarnecki A, K, Francis A, and . Jassal D (2009): Relation of biomarkers and cardiac magnetic resonance imaging after marathon running, Am J Cardiol 103.

Naylor L, Arnolda L , Deague J, Playford D , Maurogiovanni J and Green D.(2005): Reduced ventricular flow propagation velocity in elite athletes is augmented with the resumption of exercise training. J Physiol. March 15; 563(Pt 3): 957–963.

Naylor L, George K, Driscolli G and Green D (2008): The Athlete's Heart A Contemporary Appraisal of the 'Morganroth Hypothesis'. Sports Med 2008; 38 (1): 69-90.

Nistri S, Olivotto I,and Betocchi S (2006): Prognostic significance of left atrial size in patients with hypertrophic cardiomyopathy (from the Italian Registry for Hypertrophic Cardiomyopathy). Am J Cardiol 2006; 98:960–5.

Nottin S, Nguyen LD and Obert P (2004): Left ventricular function in endurance-trained children by tissue Doppler imaging. Med Sci Sports Exerc; 36:1507–13.

Ommen SR and Nishimura RA (2003): A clinical approach to the assessment of left ventricular diastolic function by doppler echocardiography. update Heart 89, iii 18-iii23.

Pasman WJ, Saris WH, Muls E, Vansant G and Westerterp-Plantenga MS (1999): Effect of exercise training on long-term weight maintenance in weight-reduced men. Metabolism. 1999 Jan;48 (1):15-21.

Pelliccia A and Maron BJ (2004): The athlete's heart, ECG, and differential diagnosis with hypertrophic cardiomyopathy and other cardiomyopathies. In: Maron BJ, editor. Diagnosis and management of hypertrophic cardiomyopathy. Malden, MA: Blackwell Futura;. p. 367–81.

Pelliccia A, Avelar E, De Castro S,and Pandian N (2000): Global left ventricular shape is not altered as a consequence of physiologic remodeling in highly trained athletes. Am J Cardiol; 86:700–2.

Pelliccia A, Culasso F and Di Paolo F (1999): Physiologic left ventricular cavity dilatation in elite athletes. Ann Intern Med; 130:23–31.

Pelliccia A, Culasso F, Di Paolo F and Maron B (1999): Physiologic left ventricular cavity dilatation in elite athletes. Ann Intern Med. 1999;130:23–31.

Pelliccia A, Fagard R, Bjørnstad HH, Anestassakis A, Arbustini E,Assanelli D, Biffi A, Borjesson M, Carrè F, Corrado D, Delise P, Dorwarth U, Hirth A, Heidbuchel H,

Hoffmann E, Mellwig KP,Panhuyzen-Goedkoop N, Pisani A, Solberg E, van-Buuren F and Vanhees L (2005): A European Society of Cardiology consensus document: recommendations for competitive sports participation in athletes with cardiovascular disease. Eur Heart J.; 26:1422–1445.

Pelliccia A, Maron BJ and Di Paolo F (2005): Prevalence and clinical significance of left atrial remodelling in competitive athletes. J Am Coll Cardiol; 46:690–6.

Pelliccia A, Maron BJ, and Di Paolo FM (2005): Prevalence and clinical significance of left atrial remodeling in competitive athletes. J Am Coll Cardiol 2005; 46:690–6.

Pelliccia A, Maron BJ, De Luca R, Di Paolo FM, Spataro A,and Culasso F (2002): Remodeling of left ventricular hypertrophy in elite athletes after long term deconditioning. Circulation; 105:944–9.

Pluim BM, Swenne CA and Zwinderman AH (1999): Correlation of heart rate variability with cardiac functional and metabolic variables in cyclists with training induced left ventricular hypertrophy. Heart; 81:612–7.

Pluim BM, Zwinderman AH and Van der Laarse A (2000): Current perspective of the athlete's heart. A meta-analysis of cardiac structure and function. Circulation; 100:336–44.

Pollock M, Gaesser G and Butcher J (1998): The recommended quantity and quality of exercise for developing and maintaining cardiorespiratory and muscular fitness and flexibility in healthy adults: American College of Sports Medicine Position Stand,. Med Sci Sports Exerc 30(6):975–991.

Popovic D, Ostojic M, Petrovic M, Vujisic-Tesic B, Popovic B, Nedeljkovic I, ArandjelovicA, Jakovljevic B, Stojanov V and Damjanovic S (2011): Assessment of the Left Ventricular Chamber Stiffness in Athletes. Echocardiography Volume 28, Issue 3, March 2011, Pages: 276–287.

Rajiv C, Vinereanu D,and Fraser AG (2004): Tissue Doppler imaging for the evaluation of patients with hypertrophic cardiomyopathy. Curr Opin Cardiol; 19:430–6.

Ranković G, Mutavdžić V, Toskić D, Preljević A, Kocić M and Damjanović N (2010): Aerobic capacity as an indicator in different kinds of sports. Bosnian journal of basic medical sciences; 10 (1): 44-48.

Rawlins J, Bhan A, and Sharma S. (2009): Left ventricular hypertrophy in athletes. European Journal of Echocardiography

10, 350–356.

Reilly T (2007): The science of training – soccer: A scientific approach to developing strength, speed and endurance. London: Routledge.

Richand V, Lafitte S, and Reant P (2007): An ultrasound speckle tracking (two-dimensional strain) analysis of myocardial deformation in professional soccer players compared with healthy subjects and hypertrophic cardiomyopathy. Am J Cardiol , 100:128–32.

Rodrigues A, Costa J, Alves G, Ferreira da Silva D, Picard M, Andrade J and Mathias W (2006): Left ventricular function after exercise training in young men. AM J Cardiol Apr 1;97(7):1089-92.

Rupp J (2001): Exercise physiology: ACSM's Health Fitness Certification Review. Philadelphia, PA, Lipincott Williams.

Russo C, Jin Z, Homma S, Rundek T,. Sacco R, and Di Tullio M (2011): Effect of Obesity and Overweight on Left

Ventricular Diastolic Function. A Community-Based Study in an Elderly Cohort, journal of the American College of Cardiology Vol. 57, No. 12, 2011.

Saito K and Matushita M (2004): The contribution of left ventricular mass to maximal oxygen uptake in female college rowers. Int J Sports Med; 25:27–31.

Sharma S, Elliott PM, Whyte G, Mahon N, Virdee MS, Mist B and McKenna WJ (2000): Utility of metabolic exercise testing in distinguishing hypertrophic cardiomyopathy from physiologic left ventricular hypertrophy in athletes.J Am Coll Cardiol. 2000 Sep;36(3):864-70.

Spencer KT, Sugeng L, Lang RM (2005): Atlas of echocardiography, chapter 1 imaging protocols and normal measurements.

Spirito P, Pelliccia A, Proschan MA, Granata M, Spataro A, and Bellone P. (1994): Morphology of the ''athlete's heart'' assessed by echocardiography in 947 elite athletes representing 27 sports. Am J Cardiol; 74:802-6.

190

Stephens M, O'Connor F and Deuster P (2002): Exercise and nutrition: AAFP Home Study—a self-assessment program. American Academy of Family Physicians, Leawood, KS.

Stewart K , Ouyang P, Bacher A, Lima S and Shapiro E (2006): Exercise effects on cardiac size and left ventricular diastolic function: relationships to changes in fitness, fatness, blood pressure and insulin resistance. Heart 2006;92:893–898.

Stolear JC, Georges B, Shita A and Verbeelen D (1999) : The predictive value of cardiac troponin t measurements in subjects on regular haemodialysis. Nephrol dial transplant (14).1961-1967.

Teare D (1958): Asymmetrical hypertrophy of the heart in young adults. Br Heart J 1958; 20:1–8.

Thomas LR and Douglas PS (2001): Echocardiographic findings in athletes. In: Thompson PD, ed. Exercise and sports cardiology.New York: McGraw-Hill,:43–70.

Thomson P and Etes M (2007): Textbook of cardiovascular medicine, Chapter 37 athletes heart , page 692.

191

Tumuklu M, Ildizli M, Ceyhan K and Cinar C (2007): Alterations in Left Ventricular Structure and Diastolic Function in Professional Football Players: Assessment by Tissue Doppler Imaging and Left Ventricular Flow Propagation Velocity. Echocardiography, Volume 24, February 2007.

Tung CL, Hsieh CK, Bien CW, and Dieuaide FR (1934): The heart in ricksha pullers. A study of the effect of chronic exertion on the cardiovascular system. Am Heart J; 10:79–100.

Vaglio Jr JC, Ommen SR, Nishimura RA, Tajik AJ and Gersh BJ (2008): Clinical characteristics and outcomes of patients with hypertrophic cardiomyopathy with a latent obstruction. Am Heart J; 156: 342–7.

Van Camp SP, Bloor CM, Mueller FO, Cantu RC and Olson HG (1995): Nontraumatic sports death in high school and college athletes. Med Sci Sports Exerc.; 27:641– 647.

Vinereanu D, Florescu N and Sculthorpe N (2001): Differentiation between pathologic and physiologic left ventricular hypertrophy by tissue Doppler assessment of long-axis function in patients with hypertrophic cardiomyopathy or systemic hypertension and in athletes. Am J Cardiol; 88:53–8.

Vinereanu D, Florescu N, Sculthorpe N, Tweddel A, Stephens M and Fraser A (2002): Left ventricular long-axis diastolic function is augmented in the hearts of endurance-trained compared with strength-trained athletes. Clinical Science (2002) 103, 249–257.

Wackerhage H, Atherton P, Babraj J and Smith K (2005): Selective activation of AMPK-PGC1a or PKB-TSC2-mTOR signaling can explain specific adaptive responses to endurance or resistance training-like electrical muscle stimulation. FASEB Journal, 19, 786–788.

Watkins H, Seidman CE, MacRae C, Seidman JG and McKenna W (1992): Progress in familial hypertrophic cardiomyopathy: molecular genetic analyses in the original family studied by Teare. Br Heart J; 67:34–8.

Whaley M and Kaminsky L (2001): Epidemiology of physical activity, physical fitness and selected chronic diseases : ACSM's Resource Manual for Guidelines for Exercise Testing and Prescription. Philadephia, PA, Lipincott Williams & Wilkins.

193

White PD (1951): Heart disease. 4th Edition. New York: MacMillan Co.; p. 612.

White PD (1951): Heart disease. 4th Edition. New York: MacMillan Co.; 1951. p. 611.

Whyte GP, George K and Middleton N (2007): Training induced changes in maximum heart rate. Int J Sports Med 2007; 28: 1-5.

Wilhelm M, Brem M, Rost C , Klinghammer L and Flachskampf F (2010): Early Repolarization, Left Ventricular Diastolic Function, and Left Atrial Size in Professional Soccer Players The American Journal of Cardiology, Volume 106, Issue 4, 15 August Pages 569-574.

Wilmore H (2003): The science of exercise physiology: Aerobic exercise and endurance. Phys. Sportsmed. 31(May):45–51.

Wilmore JH and Costill DL. (2005): Physiology of Sport and Exercise: 3rd Edition. Champaign, IL: Human Kinetics.

Wygand J (2001): Exercise programming: ACSM's Health Fitness Certification Review.Philadelphia, PA, Lippincott Williams & Wilkins.

Youngblood D (2005): The beat goes on. Minneapolis Star Tribune. December 18, Sports section: 10.

Ziya S, Fuat G, Sertac A, Zinnur G, and, Sule K (2011): Analysis of athletes' heart by tissue Doppler and strain/strain rate imaging. The International Journal of Cardiovascular Imaging, Volume 27, Number 1, January 2011 , pp. 105-111(7).

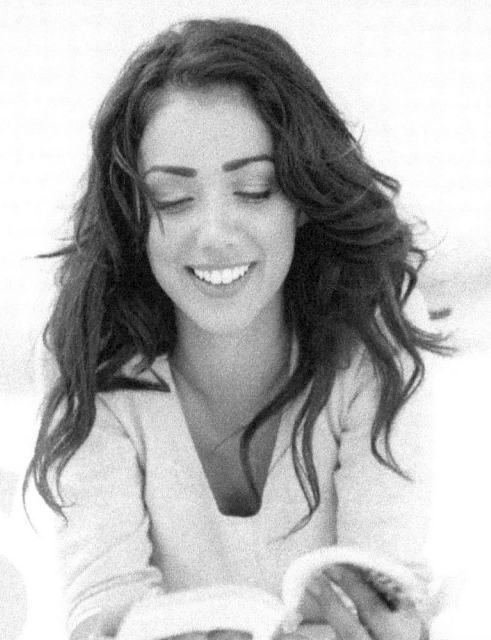
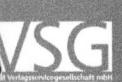